CAMBRIDGE STUDIES IN PHILOSOPHY

Sensations

CAMBRIDGE STUDIES IN PHILOSOPHY

General editor SYDNEY SHOEMAKER

Advisory editors J. E. J. ALTHAM, SIMON BLACKBURN,
GILBERT HARMAN, MARTIN HOLLIS, FRANK JACKSON,
JONATHAN LEAR, WILLIAM LYCAN, JOHN PERRY, BARRY STROUD

Sensations

A DEFENSE OF TYPE MATERIALISM

Christopher S. Hill

University of Arkansas, Fayetteville

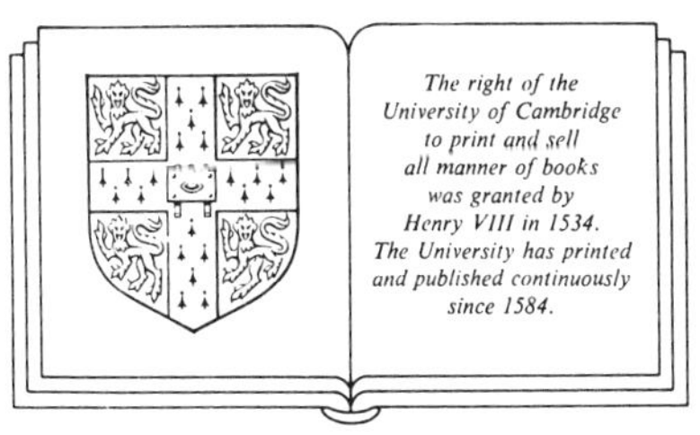

Cambridge University Press

Cambridge

New York   Port Chester   Melbourne   Sydney

Published by the Press Syndicate of the University of Cambridge
The Pitt Building, Trumpington Street, Cambridge CB2 1RP
40 West 20th Street, New York, NY 10011, USA
10 Stamford Road, Oakleigh, Melbourne 3166, Australia

© Cambridge University Press 1991

First published 1991

Printed in the United States of America

Library of Congress Cataloging-in-Publication Data
Hill, Christopher S.
Sensations : a defense of type materialism / Christopher S. Hill.
p.   cm. – (Cambridge studies in philosophy)
Includes index.
ISBN 0-521-39423-6 (hardcover). – ISBN 0-521-39737-5 (pbk.)
1. Senses and sensation.   2. Knowledge, Theory of.   I. Title.
II. Title: Type materialism.   III. Series.
BD214.H54   1991
128′.3 – dc 20   90-15019
                                                             CIP

British Library Cataloging-in-Publication Data
applied for.

ISBN 0 521 394236 hardback
ISBN 0 521 397375 paperback

For my parents
Martha Van Schelven Hill
William Surleau Hill

Contents

Preface   *page* ix

PART ONE: INTRODUCTION   1

1   Topics and themes   3

PART TWO: THE MIND–BODY PROBLEM   17

2   The failings of dualism and the double-aspect theory   19
3   The failings of functionalism   44
4   In defense of type materialism   83

PART THREE: INTROSPECTION   115

5   Introspective awareness of sensations   117
6   Introspection and the skeptic   139

PART FOUR: SENSORY CONCEPTS   157

7   Concepts of bodily sensations: Their semantic properties   159
8   Concepts of visual sensations: Their content and their deployment   186

PART FIVE: OTHER MINDS   207

9   Knowledge of other minds   209
10   Unity of consciousness, other minds, and phenomenal space   228

Index   245

Preface

I am quite interested in winning new friends for the views that this book
defends – as many new friends as possible. Accordingly, I have written
for a group that is somewhat more inclusive than the community of
professional philosophers. I hope the book will find readers among
undergraduate philosophy students and also among computer scientists,
neuroscientists, and psychologists. (Some readers may find that the
second half of Chapter 2 and the middle of Chapter 3 are a bit taxing. I
hope they will persevere. A partial understanding of this material is
entirely sufficient for an adequate grasp of the main themes of the book.)

My main debts are to Ivan Fox and Sydney Shoemaker, each of whom has
been extremely generous with his time and wisdom. They have saved me
from many errors, and pointed the way toward many ideas that would
otherwise have eluded me. Although it is somewhat paradoxical, since
they both disagree with many of my main contentions, it is nonetheless
true that such value as the book may have is largely due to them.

I have received encouragement and valuable help of other kinds from
Anthony L. Brueckner, Anil Gupta, Richard Lee, William G. Lycan,
R.J. Nelson, Hilary Putnam, Vola Shulkin, Lynne Spellman, and Chris
Swoyer. Each has played an important role at several stages. I am also
indebted to Clyde L. Hardin and Brian McLaughlin, who commented
on the penultimate draft. In addition, I have benefited significantly
from technical assistance provided by Maggie Blades, Karen Carroll,
Ronald Cohen, and Linda Morgan. And I have received more limited –
but nonetheless extremely useful – assistance from a number of other
associates. They are thanked by name in footnotes.

Financial support from the National Endowment for the Humanities
continues to be remembered with gratitude, as does an Off-Campus
Duty Assignment from the University of Arkansas. Finally, I take
pleasure in recording a deep debt to the National Humanities Center,
which provided me with an ideal environment during the academic
year 1987–1988.

PART ONE

Introduction

1

Topics and themes

In these pages we will be concerned with sensations themselves (that is, with concrete sensory events) and also with certain of the characteristics that sensations exemplify. Although we will consider characteristics of other kinds as well, we will be primarily concerned with characteristics that are *qualitative*. Qualitative characteristics include *being a pain* and *being an itch*. They also include the sensory characteristic that is exemplified by the gustatory sensations one has when one tastes orange juice, and the sensory characteristic that is exemplified by the olfactory sensations one has when one smells gasoline.[1]

A terminological point. Ordinary language does not contain many names for qualitative characteristics of sensations (or *qualia*, as I shall sometimes call them). In addition to *"being a pain"* there is *"being an itch"* and *"being a case of pleasure."* But there are not many others. In most cases we pick out qualitative characteristics of sensations by resorting to descriptions, and this is what I have done in giving the last two examples in the first paragraph. However, it can seem that descriptions like "the sensory characteristic that is exemplified by the gustatory sensations one has when one tastes orange juice" suffer from crippling ambiguities. If, for example, one tastes orange juice right after brushing one's teeth with mint flavored toothpaste, one experiences a sensa-

1 At this point it is best to explain "qualitative" by appealing to examples; to do otherwise would prejudge an important metaphysical question about the nature of qualitative characteristics.

In using the term "qualitative," I mean to single out the class of characteristics that includes *being a pain, being an itch*, and all others of the same metaphysical type. As I see it, the most salient common features of the members of this class are, first, that they are intrinsic characteristics, and second, that they determine membership in sensory kinds. Hence, if I were asked to define the notion of a qualitative characteristic, I would give a definition that was based on these two features. On the other hand, most philosophers who favor the view known as functionalism would wish to deny that *being a pain* can appropriately be described as an intrinsic characteristic. For this reason, it seems best to work with a loose and intuitive conception of a qualitative characteristic until we have examined functionalism. After Chapter 3, which is devoted to functionalism, we will be in a position to adopt a definition of the sort just mentioned.

tion – a most unpleasant sensation – that is quite different than the one that is normally associated with tasting orange juice. And one has a sensation of yet another kind when one tastes orange juice right after drinking scotch. And so on. In view of these considerations it seems that the foregoing description fails to pick out a unique qualitative characteristic. Evidently, in order to guard against this ambiguity, it is necessary to use a more elaborate description – a description like "the sensory characteristic that is exemplified by the gustatory sensations that a normal person has when he or she tastes orange juice under standard perceptual conditions."

Perhaps I have not yet added enough qualifications to eliminate all ambiguities. After all, what counts as a normal person varies from possible world to possible world, and the perceptual conditions that count as standard in one world tend to be different than the conditions that count as standard in other worlds. We can, for example, imagine a possible world in which human nervous systems are sufficiently different that the normal taste of orange juice is quite different than it is in the actual world. Accordingly, one might think that even a complicated description like the one cited at the end of the last paragraph stands ambiguously for the members of a set of qualia, one for each of the possible worlds that is relevantly different from ours. So perhaps it is necessary to make use of certain very complicated descriptions – descriptions like "the sensory characteristic that is exemplified by the gustatory sensations that a normal person has when he or she tastes orange juice under conditions that are standard in the actual world."

I

When we approach sensations and their qualitative characteristics from a theoretical perspective, we encounter a number of questions that either have a philosophical dimension or fall entirely within the purview of philosophy. Most of these questions can be assigned to one of the following five categories.

1. QUASI-EMPIRICAL QUESTIONS

Is there an interesting correspondence or dependency relationship between qualitative characteristics and physical characteristics of some sort?

Take, for example, the relationship of *universal correlation* – the relationship that would obtain between a qualitative characteristic and a physical characteristic if it were true that, for any being x, x experiences a token of the qualitative characteristic when and only when a token of the physical characteristic occurs in x's brain. Is there a set of physical characteristics that are universally correlated with the set of qualitative characteristics?

Questions about correspondence and dependency relationships between qualitative and physical characteristics are quasi-empirical rather than purely empirical because they presuppose answers to certain questions about the distribution of sensations – questions that cannot be adequately answered on the basis of empirical information alone.

Thus, suppose that pain is distributed quite broadly. Specifically, suppose that it would be correct to ascribe pains to certain androids whose brains differ from ours both in structure and in material composition. (Suppose that the pain-behavior of these androids is indistinguishable from ours. Suppose also – probably contrary to fact – that a similarity of this sort counts as a sufficient reason for ascribing pain to other beings.) Suppose further that there is one and only one physical state-type whose instances are correlated with pain in human beings, and that the internal differences between ourselves and the androids are sufficiently great that it is obviously wrong to say that this state-type is exemplified by any of the events that take place in the brains of the androids. Clearly, in combination with these latter assumptions, our assumption about the correctness of ascribing pain to these androids implies that there is no physical state-type whose instances are universally correlated with pains.

To settle questions about the distribution of sensations it is not enough to conduct an empirical investigation. Empirical inquiry can give us all the information we might like to have about the behavior and nervous systems of, say, earthworms, but unsupplemented empirical inquiry cannot settle the question of whether earthworms can experience pain. Nor can it tell us whether shrimps, or crickets, or silicon-based androids can feel pain. To determine how widely pain is distributed we must first determine what counts as an adequate reason for ascribing a sensory state to a being other than oneself. We must obtain a list of criteria that can be used to distinguish between ascriptions that are legitimate and ascriptions that are not, and we must assign appropriate weights to the criteria on the list. The task of drawing up a list of this sort falls within the province of philosophy. It is not a scientific task.

2. METAPHYSICAL QUESTIONS

What is the ultimate nature of sensory events? Are they ultimately physical in nature or do they belong to a nonphysical realm?

Materialists maintain that we obtain a simpler and more straightforward picture of the universe if we assume that sensory events are identical with physical events. We are obliged to make this assumption, they contend, because we have a general duty of reason to refrain from multiplying entities beyond necessity, and because we have a duty of reason to prefer theories that are clear and informative to theories that are obscure and sketchy. (It has generally been assumed by materialists that if we deny that sensory events are identical with physical events, we will not be able to give an illuminating account of the connections between them. We may be able to say that they are connected by causal ties, but it will prove impossible to give an intellectually satisfying account of the nature of these ties.)

On the other hand, dualists have called attention to a number of obstacles to identifying sensory events with physical events, some of which are quite serious. One of these obstacles can be expressed by saying that the relationship between sensations and physical events seems to be similar to the relationship that obtains between the lights one sees when one views a city at night, and the dark spaces that lie between the lights. Sensations are colorful and luminous; physical events are colorless, dark, and lifeless. Accordingly, dualists claim, they cannot be the same. Another obstacle derives from the fact that the connections between sensory events and physical events can seem to be radically contingent. This obstacle is captured by the following Cartesian argument:

> **First premise.** Conceivability is an adequate test for possibility. That is to say, if we can clearly and distinctly conceive of its being the case that p, then it is genuinely possible for it to be the case that p.

> **Second premise.** Where x is any sensory event and y is any physical event (even one that materialists might claim to be identical with x), it is possible to conceive clearly and distinctly of x occurring without being accompanied by y, and it is possible to conceive clearly and distinctly of y occurring without being accompanied by x.

> **Third premise.** If it is possible for an entity to exist without being accompanied by a second entity, the first entity cannot be identical with the second.

> **Conclusion.** Sensory events are not identical with physical events.

It may be that materialism is capable of surmounting or circumventing these two obstacles, and also all of the other obstacles that dualists have pointed out. But this is not obvious. There is a case for dualism that is prima facie quite strong.

In addition to asking about the ultimate metaphysical nature of sensory events, it is necessary to ask about the ultimate nature of qualitative characteristics.

There are at least three answers to this second question that deserve to be taken seriously. One answer asserts that qualia are identical with straightforwardly physical characteristics – that is, with characteristics that things have by virtue of their physical structure and/or their material composition. The second answer begins by explaining the notion of a functional characteristic. Very roughly speaking, a characteristic is functional if (1) it is exemplifiable by certain of the internal states of a system, and (2) the internal states that exemplify it do so purely by virtue of their causal and counterfactual relations to inputs, to outputs, and to other internal states. According to the second answer, qualitative characteristics are identical with certain functional characteristics. The third answer is the one that is favored by dualists. It claims that qualia cannot be reduced either to physical characteristics or to functional characteristics. Qualia comprise a third realm of characteristics, a realm whose constituents cannot be fully grasped by the sort of analytical techniques that are used in the sciences. Rather, they can be fully grasped only by being felt or experienced.

Although materialism has in the twentieth century come to replace dualism in the affections of philosophers, we do not yet have an unanswerable justification for this preference. Nor do we have an adjudication of the dispute among the three schools of thought about qualitative characteristics. Thus, even after centuries of discussion, the main metaphysical questions about sensations and their qualitative characteristics are open.

Preserving what I believe to be the main strand in the history of its use, I will employ the term "mind–body problem" as a label for these questions.

3. EPISTEMOLOGICAL QUESTIONS

What is the nature of introspective awareness of sensations? Is there an "inner eye" – some sort of scanning device that can sweep across the sensory firmament and zoom in on particular items that are of interest for one reason or another? If not, what alternative theory should we accept?

What is the epistemological status of our beliefs about sensations? Many philosophers have claimed certainty and incorrigibility for our introspective beliefs. Are these claims correct? If so, how can we explain this fact? And if not, what degree of reliability should we assign to introspection? Should we say, with many contemporary psychologists, that introspection is completely untrustworthy? Should we abandon the view, held by William James and many nineteenth-century psychologists, that introspection is capable of playing a useful role in the scientific study of the mind?

Are we omniscient about our sensations, as many philosophers have claimed? When a sensation occurs, is its owner inevitably aware of it – at least to some degree? Or are there sensations that lie beyond our ken?

Finally, although it has generally been assumed that it is impossible to raise systemic doubts about our beliefs concerning sensations that parallel the familiar skeptical doubts about our beliefs concerning the external world, this assumption has never received a fully adequate defense. Is the assumption correct? If it is, why?

4. SEMANTIC QUESTIONS

How do our sensory concepts acquire their contents? And what is the nature of their contents?

It has often been held that sensory concepts acquire their contents from internal ostensive definitions, and that their contents are largely or entirely ostensive (in the sense that the question of whether one is entitled to apply a sensory concept to a given sensation depends largely or entirely on the immediate qualitative nature of the sensation). The appeal of this position is obvious. We are all inclined to say that it is possible for someone to determine correctly whether a sensory concept applies to one of his or her own sensations simply by focusing introspectively on its qualitative characteristics.

An alternative view asserts that the contents of our sensory concepts derive from the roles they play in a commonsense psychological theory. According to this view, we cannot be said to have acquired a concept of pain until we know some facts about the typical causes and effects of pain. We must know, among other things, that pain is typically caused by bodily damage or by dangerous extremes of temperature and pressure, and that pain typically causes crying and various forms of avoidance behavior. Like the first view, this view can seem highly attractive.

There are a number of other views about the contents of our sensory concepts, several of which enjoy at least as much prima facie plausibility as the two I have already cited.

Which of these views should be accepted? And on what grounds?

5. QUESTIONS ABOUT OTHER MINDS

In addition to the foregoing epistemological questions about introspective awareness of one's own sensations, there are several extremely difficult epistemological questions concerning beliefs about the sensations of others. Can one appropriately claim to know that other human beings have sensations? If so, can one appropriately claim to know that they have sensations that are much like one's own? Further, can one appropriately claim to know that members of other biological species have sensations? If so, which species? And which sensations? How far can one proceed down the evolutionary scale before it becomes inappropriate to ascribe sensations? And what about androids?

There are also some important metaphysical questions about other minds. Consider these two situations: In the first, I am feeling a pain and experiencing the taste of orange juice; in the second, I am feeling a pain and *you* are experiencing the taste of orange juice. What is the difference between these situations? That is, in what does the otherness of your sensations consist? In general, what is the difference between a situation in which two sensations belong to a single state of consciousness (or a single sensory field) and a situation in which two sensations belong to two different states of consciousness (or two different sensory fields)? That is to say, what is the nature of unity of consciousness?

II

The questions I have been reviewing are the main topics of this work. In the hope that doing so will enhance the accessibility of later chapters, I will now provide a brief summary of the positions I will take in responding to them.

1. At this point in time it would be premature to attempt to answer the quasi-empirical questions. Today we are not even able to say for sure whether there is a law-like correlation between sensory states and neural states in human beings. However, there are two issues associated with the quasi-empirical questions that we *are* able to discuss.

First, we are in a position to get clearer about the criteria that are relevant to determining how widely sensations are distributed. I will show that the criteria in question are not only sensitive to behavioral and functional considerations, but to biological considerations as well. Thus, among other things, I will try to show that we are not entitled to ascribe determinate sensations to other beings unless certain biological conditions are satisfied. (If my arguments for this claim are sound, then we are not entitled to ascribe sensations to nonbiological androids. So the lines of thought that I will develop will suggest answers to *some* questions about the distribution of sensations.)

Second, we are in a position to get a bit clearer about the status of the *psychophysical correlation thesis*:

> Where ϕ is any qualitative characteristic of sensations, it is possible to find a *neural* characteristic ψ such that the following proposition about ϕ and ψ expresses a law of nature: Where x is any being whatsoever, x has a sensation that exemplifies ϕ when and only when an event that exemplifies ψ takes place in x's brain.

Although we are unable today to determine whether this thesis is fully compatible with the relevant empirical facts, I think we are in a position to clear away the objections that have convinced many contemporary philosophers that it is false. The objections are often taken to be empirical in character, but on closer examination they turn out to have an a priori dimension that makes them vulnerable to philosophical criticism. I will show that they are misguided, and that acceptance of the psychophysical correlation thesis is therefore a live option.

Other correlation theses might be considered. In fact, where K is any category of physical characteristics such that there is a one-to-one mapping between the category of qualitative characteristics and the members of K, there is a correlation thesis that claims that each member of the category of qualitative characteristics is universally correlated with its image in K. In this work, however, I will set all other correlation theses aside and focus on the one that is formulated in the preceding paragraph, for it is more in keeping than the others with my view that other beings must satisfy certain biological conditions before it can be reasonable for one to ascribe sensations to them.

No single part of this book is devoted to the members of the family of quasi-empirical questions. Most of what I have to say about them can be found in Part 2 and Part 5, but there are also some relevant arguments in Part 4.

2. In order to summarize my answers to the metaphysical questions, I must first distinguish between two forms of materialism.

Token materialism is the view that results from combining the proposition that every sensory event is identical with some physical event with the proposition that the characteristics by virtue of which events count as sensory are numerically distinct from the characteristics by virtue of which they count as physical (that is, with the proposition that qualitative characteristics are not identical with physical characteristics of any kind). Token materialism does not presuppose the existence of a universal correlation between sensory characteristics and physical characteristics, and it is therefore compatible with the possibility of there being two or more events of the same sensory type that are respectively identical with events that are of quite different physical types.[2] On the other hand, a token materialist does not deny the existence of a universal correlation. Token materialism is largely free from commitments concerning quasi-empirical issues.

Type materialism is like token materialism in claiming that sensory events are identical with physical events. However, it also claims that there is a set of physical characteristics with which qualitative characteristics are universally and lawfully correlated, and that every qualitative characteristic is identical with its physical correlate. As this description shows, type materialists have a certain amount of latitude. One option is to embrace the psychophysical correlation thesis and assert that qualitative characteristics are identical with the neural characteristics that this thesis claims to be correlated with them. However, it is also quite possible for type materialists to take a different line. They can deny that qualitative characteristics are correlated with neural characteristics and maintain that they are correlated instead with physical characteristics of some other sort. They can then

---

2 Here and elsewhere, when I speak of a correlation between sensory characteristics and physical characteristics, I mean a correlation between sensory universals and physical universals. (Roughly speaking, universals are characteristics that are responsible for the objective resemblances and the causal powers of particulars. See David Lewis, "New Work for a Theory of Universals," *Australasian Journal of Philosophy* 61 (1983), pp. 343–77. See also Lewis, *On the Plurality of Worlds* (Oxford: Blackwell, 1986), pp. 50–69. (Although the sense that Lewis assigns to the term "universal" corresponds pretty closely to the sense that I wish to assign to it here, it turns out that the closest Lewisian counterpart of "universal," as I wish to use it, is "natural property." See "New Work for a Theory of Universals," pp. 346–47.) I use "state-type" as an equivalent of "universal.")

go on to identify qualitative characteristics with these other physical characteristics.

Alas, for reasons that are not entirely clear to me, type materialism does not have many friends in the contemporary philosophical community. Indeed, it is one of the least popular theories in philosophy of mind, if not all of philosophy. However, in my judgment, it deserves to be taken seriously, and it may well represent the correct answer to the mind–body problem. I will defend this view in Part 2. In constructing my defense I will concentrate on the version of type materialism that presupposes the truth of the psychophysical correlation thesis. This will, I hope, make the issues a bit more vivid. Also, because I find the psychophysical correlation thesis more plausible than other members of the family of correlation theses (see the penultimate paragraph of section III.1), this version of the theory is closer to my heart than other versions. I am much more interested in making a case for the proposition that *it* may be correct than in making a case for the proposition that some version or other may be correct.

After Part 2, type materialism will no longer be in the foreground. However, it will not disappear from view. In discussing the other questions about sensations, I will show that they have answers that are fully compatible with the preferred version of type materialism.

3. According to the Cartesian picture of mind, our epistemic access to our sensations is like God's epistemic access to the physical world. First, awareness of sensations is immediate: There is no medium through which sensations are apprehended, nor does awareness of sensations involve representations or appearances of any kind. There is no "epistemic distance" between the inner eye and the sensations to which it attends. Second, our beliefs about our sensations are infallible. When, for example, it seems to a subject that he or she is in pain, then he or she really is in pain. And third, each of us is omniscient with respect to his or her sensations. The field of vision of one's inner eye encompasses one's entire sensory realm, and this eye is able to apprehend details with microscopic accuracy.

These views have been anathema to most twentieth-century psychologists and to a great many twentieth-century philosophers working in the analytical tradition. Beginning with the early behaviorists, introspection has been the target of an unremitting and many-pronged attack. Among other things, it has been charged that the deliverances of introspection are distorted by influences of various kinds (e.g., expectations), that the concepts used in forming beliefs about sensations suffer from an unacceptably high degree of vagueness, that these concepts presuppose a large number of radically false beliefs about the nature of sensations and the nature of their relations to one another and to other things, and that it is impossible even to determine the degree of unreliability of introspection because experimental inquiries about introspection are not subject to the constraints associated with intersubjective checking. Even today, long after the overthrow of behaviorism, worries of this sort are widespread. There is no place in psychology for experiments based on introspection, and philosophers tend to feel little affection for the Cartesian epistemological tradition.

I will chart a course between these familiar positions. It seems to me that contemporary worries about introspection are partly due to the fact that we do not have even a remotely adequate grasp of what it is that introspection is supposed to be. Accordingly, I will devote more attention than is customary among philosophers to quasi-empirical questions about the nature of introspection. The view that I wish to recommend is a two-factor theory that results from splicing together two different metaphors. The theory postulates an internal scanner that has some of the properties of the human eye, and also claims that introspection has components that are like the processes of adjusting the tuning and turning up the volume on a radio.

Concerning questions about the epistemic status of introspective beliefs, I will argue that there is an important sense in which Cartesian claims of immediacy are correct. Recognition of this fact enables us to see that contemporary doubts about the deliverances of introspection are partially misguided. However, I hold no brief for the Cartesian claims that we are infallible or omniscient with respect to our sensations, and I will in fact try to strengthen some of the objections that have been raised against them.

In addition to sketching a theory of the nature of introspection and offering a qualified defense of Cartesianism, I will discuss the question of whether it is possible to develop a skeptical argument about introspective awareness that would be the counterpart of the familiar skeptical arguments about knowledge of external objects. Is it possible for an evil genius to deceive us systematically about the existence and/or nature of sensations? I will try to justify a negative answer to this question.

4. Questions about the contents of sensory concepts have important connections with metaphysical questions about sensations. Indeed, the question of whether it is appropriate for us to accept type materialism depends on our disposition of certain semantic issues.

In order that we may better appreciate this point, let us take another look at the second of the two views we considered in connection with the semantic questions in the previous section. According to this view, which might be called the *implicit definition theory*, the contents of our sensory concepts derive from the roles that the concepts play in our commonsense theory of mental activity – the concepts are implicitly defined by the laws of the theory. Now it is reasonable to suppose that the laws of the theory in question link our sensory concepts to concepts of three different kinds – to concepts that stand for various types of stimulation, to concepts that stand for various types of behavior, and to concepts that stand for various types of nonsensory internal state. Accordingly, the implicit definition theory implies that the contents of our sensory concepts are internally linked to the contents of our concepts of these other three kinds. It implies, for example, that it is part of the concept of pain that pain is normally caused by damage to the body or by a bodily disturbance of some kind, that pain normally causes wincing and crying out, and that it also normally causes distress and the desire to seek relief.

Now if the implicit definition theory is correct, then every type of sensation is associated with a certain causal role, and the causal role that is associated with a given type of sensation is constitutive of what it is to be a sensation of that type. But this implies that it would be a mistake to identify types of sensation with types of neural state. For the nature of a neural state depends entirely on the properties of its constituent neurons and the relations they bear to one another, not on the causal role that the state plays in some larger biological system. It follows that the implicit definition theory is incompatible with type materialism.

For this reason, and for other reasons, it is incumbent on me to provide an alternative to the implicit definition theory. As I see it, any reasonable alternative must incorporate elements from one or both of the following views. First, there is the view that sensory concepts get their contents from internal ostensive definitions, and that their contents are therefore largely or entirely ostensive in nature. (This view is of course the first of the two positions we considered in section II.) Second, there is the view that sensory concepts acquire their reference from causal descriptions of the form "the state-type that plays such-and-such causal role in beings of type T," but that they are not synonymous with such descriptions. Instead of claiming that causal descriptions *define* our sensory concepts, this view asserts only that the

14

former are used to *fix the reference* of the latter. Accordingly, it does not imply that there are internal relations between sensory concepts and concepts of causal roles. (Readers of Kripke's *Naming and Necessity* will have recognized that the second view owes much to his ideas.[3] According to Kripke, it is possible to use a description to assign a referent to a term or a concept without thereby making the term or concept synonymous with the description. When this happens, one is said to have used the description to fix the reference of the term or concept.)

In Part 4 I will recommend a position that can be described as a compromise between these two views and the implicit definition theory. This position claims that we have a set of sensory concepts that are largely or entirely ostensive, and that we also have a set whose members acquire their reference from causal descriptions by the process of reference-fixing. In addition to making these claims, it asserts that causal descriptions are built into the contents of some of our sensory concepts. This last claim is of course a concession to the intuitions that underlie the implicit definition theory, but as it turns out, it is not a concession that has serious implications for type materialism.

5. In discussing epistemological questions about other minds, I will argue for the view that a combination of behavioral and biological factors can make it reasonable for one to ascribe determinate sensations to other beings. Also, as mentioned earlier, I will defend the view that we are not entitled to make such ascriptions unless certain biological conditions are satisfied. In arguing for the first view I will rehabilitate the traditional argument from analogy. More specifically, I will show that one is justified in reasoning as follows: Sensations of certain kinds mediate between stimuli and responses of various kinds in my own case; the members of group G are sensitive to more or less the same stimuli as I am, and they tend to respond to these stimuli in more or less the same ways; moreover, the members of group G belong to the same biological kind as I do (or to a related biological kind); so it is likely that the members of G have sensations like my own. In arguing for the second view, I will maintain that we must recognize that there are biological constraints on the enterprise of ascribing sensations if we are to avoid making ascriptions that seem on reflection to be misguided or even absurd.

3 See Saul A. Kripke, *Naming and Necessity* (Cambridge, MA: Harvard University Press, 1980), 53–60.

In discussing the 'otherness' of other minds (that is, the metaphysical question of how the unity of consciousness is to be analyzed), I will show that philosophers have erred in viewing unity of consciousness as a single phenomenon. Contrary to what is often maintained, the sensory field is held together by a number of overlapping relations – relations that tend to have little or nothing in common.

These lines of thought about other minds will be found in Part 5.

PART TWO

The mind–body problem

2

The failings of dualism
and the double-aspect theory

My goal in Part 2 is to convince the reader that type materialism deserves to be taken seriously. I will work toward this goal by establishing three propositions. First, in this chapter I will show that, under certain assumptions, type materialism is to be preferred to two of its most significant rivals – dualism and a view that is often called the *double-aspect theory*. Second, in the next chapter, I will argue for the proposition that its other main rival, a view known as *functionalism*, suffers from serious defects. And finally, two chapters hence, I will establish that the main objections to type materialism are misguided.

I

When J.J.C. Smart and other materialists of the 1950s and early 1960s set out to defend their favorite doctrines, they were typically more concerned to answer objections than to construct positive supporting arguments. It seems to have been generally felt that materialism has a certain intrinsic plausibility that competing theories lack, and that as a result, once the objections to materialism were answered, the burden of proof would shift to the shoulders of the advocates of other theories. Thus, instead of giving carefully formulated positive arguments, the materialists of Smart's era relied mainly on sketchy appeals to simplicity and terse complaints about the obscurity and messiness of competing views.[1]

Much of section I of this chapter is excerpted from my paper, "In Defense of Type Materialism" (*Synthese* 59 (1984), 295–320). The rest was written while I was a participant in Michael Resnik's N.E.H. seminar in the summer of 1988. I have benefited from Resnik's comments on an earlier version.

1 In the 1950s it was fashionable to accuse dualists of being committed to "nomological danglers" – a charge that certainly sounds serious! However, as far as I have been able to determine, no one ever bothered to prove that dualism has such commitments. (The term "nomological dangler" was introduced by Herbert Feigl, who used it to refer to laws that contain concepts that make no real contribution to scientific explanations.

This pattern has persisted to the present. Very little has been done to improve the arguments of the materialists of Smart's day. Moreover, while one or two new lines of thought have appeared in the literature, they have been devised with the intention of supporting token material-ism.[2] Virtually nothing has been done to add to the credentials of forms of type materialism.

In this chapter I will remedy this situation. I will show that type materialism is superior to dualism and the double-aspect theory by an argument that is based on the notion of explanatory power. In addition, I will consider the prospects of deriving a second superiority result from the simplicity-based arguments that were adumbrated by the early materialists. Finally, I will briefly consider the question of whether there is a third way of defending type materialism.

First, a few words about the content of dualism and the double-aspect theory.

As is well known, dualism comes in a variety of guises. Some dualists have asserted or presupposed the existence of a nonphysical substance – a substance they have identified with the subject or owner of mental states. Other dualists have denied the existence of such a substance, and have maintained that the self is nothing more than a set or bundle of individual mental states that are connected by ties of causation, mem-ory, similarity, and so on. Dualists have also disagreed about the existence and nature of causal relations between mental states and events in the physical world. Some have maintained that there is two-way causal interaction. Others have maintained that there is causal interaction but that it is unidirectional. Still others have maintained that the mental and the physical are causally isolated from one another.

Although the controversies that divide dualists are interesting, I wish to set them all aside. And I wish to set aside all that dualists have said about mental states other than sensations. Thus, as seen here, dualism is just a view about the metaphysical nature of sensations. For me, in this work, dualism is just the view that sensory events are not identical with

---

See Herbert Feigl, "The 'Mental' and the 'Physical'," *Minnesota Studies in the Philosophy of Science*, Vol. II (Minneapolis: University of Minnesota Press, 1958), 370–497. See, especially, p. 428.)

2 The most celebrated new argument is probably the one in Donald Davidson's "Mental Events." This essay is reprinted in Davidson's *Actions and Events* (Oxord: Oxford University Press, 1980), 207–25.

physical events (where, of course, this is taken to imply that the qualitative characteristics of sensations are not identical with physical characteristics).

As seen here, the double-aspect theory has the following three components: first, the claim that sensory events are identical with physical events; second, the doctrine that qualitative characteristics are not identical with physical characteristics; and third, the proposition that qualitative characteristics are intrinsic characteristics (in the sense that they cannot be analyzed in terms of causal powers or any other properties that entail actual or counterfactual relations between sensations and other things). Thus, according to the double-aspect theory, every sensation is both sensory and physical. Every sensation has an irreducibly sensory aspect and an irreducibly physical aspect. (As we will see later, the first two components of the double-aspect theory are also components of the standard versions of functionalism. We need the third component to keep the double-aspect theory separate from these versions.)

In arguing that dualism and the double-aspect theory are inferior to type materialism, I will assume the truth of the psychophysical correlation thesis. This is risky. As I noted earlier, the thesis at present has the status of a bold conjecture. Insofar as my arguments for the superiority of type materialism presuppose the truth of the thesis, they are in danger of being undermined by future empirical inquiry. On the other hand, I will not be begging any questions in assuming that the thesis is true. Unlike functionalism, the other chief competitor of type materialism, dualism and the double-aspect theory are entirely compatible with the thesis – compatible both in letter and in spirit. Indeed, a number of the philosophers who have been advocates of these theories have suspected that the thesis might well turn out to be correct. Further, I see no reason to believe that the risk that we incur by assuming the thesis is unacceptably large. It is true that we do not have a great deal of positive evidence for the thesis, but it is also true that such evidence is not altogether lacking. Moreover, as I will argue later, the objections that are raised against the thesis in the contemporary literature are largely without merit.

As I noted in Chaper 1, dualists have attempted to secure their own position by raising objections to type materialism. There are many such objections in the literature, and there are also a number of objections that have been raised by advocates of the double-aspect theory. In this chapter I will simply assume that the objections in these two groups can be answered. Later, in Chapter 4, I will defend this assumption by responding to several representative objections from each group.

II

The strongest reason for preferring type materialism to dualism and the double-aspect theory derives from a proposition that is sometimes called the *best explanation principle*. This proposition is in effect a rule of inductive inference. It can be formulated as follows: If a theory provides a good explanation of a set of facts, and the explanation is better than any explanation provided by a competing theory, there is a good and sufficient reason for believing that the theory is true.

As a number of authors (for example, Sellars, Harman, Lycan) have observed, it is reasonable to suppose that we are governed by this principle – that is, that it is one of the rules of ampliative inference that guide our reasoning and shape our intuitions about the inductive strength of arguments.[3] Thus, it seems necessary to suppose that we are governed by the principle in order to explain why we feel that it is rational to accept scientific theories that postulate unobservable phenomena. Moreover, as Harman has often argued, the principle seems to underlie a great deal of the ampliative reasoning that takes place in everyday life. For example, a detective may defend a hypothesis about the identity of a murderer by showing that it explains more of the facts of a case than the rival hypotheses, or by showing that it explains the facts better than its rivals.

Although the best explanation principle is not always cited by name in discussions of inductive inference, it is widely held among epistemologists and philosophers of science that the acceptability of hypotheses depends to a large extent upon their explanatory power. It is, for example, often maintained that, all else being equal, we should prefer the theory that leaves the smallest number of explanatory loose ends. Properly qualified, principles of this sort turn out to be at least roughly equivalent to the best explanation principle.[4]

---

3 See Wilfrid Sellars, *Science, Perception, and Reality* (London: Routledge and Kegan Paul, 1963); Gilbert Harman, "The Inference to the Best Explanation," *The Philosophical Review* 74 (1966), 88–95; Harman, "Knowledge, Inference, and Explanation," *American Philosophical Quarterly* 5 (1968), 164–73; Harman, *Change in View* (Cambridge, MA: MIT Press, 1987), Chapter 7; and William G. Lycan, *Judgement and Justification* (Cambridge: Cambridge University Press, 1988), Chapter 7.

4 It should be mentioned that there are philosophers who have deep reservations about the best explanation principle (see, for example, Peter Railton, "Explanation and

22

As I mentioned earlier, I wish to assume here that the psychophysical correlation thesis is correct. If I am right, the objections against it can be answered. It is not inappropriate, then, to assume tentatively that the thesis is true. Let us do so. And let us combine it with the best explanation principle. This gives us the following argument:

> **First premise.** If a theory provides a good explanation of a set of facts, and the explanation is better than any explanation provided by a competing theory, then one has a good and sufficient reason to believe that the theory is true.
>
> **Second premise.** Type materialism provides a good explanation of the psychophysical correlations that are claimed to exist by the psychophysical correlation thesis.
>
> **Third premise.** Moreover, the explanation that it provides is superior to the explanations provided by all competing theories.
>
> **Conclusion.** Provided that the psychophysical correlation thesis is true, we have good and sufficient reason to believe that type materialism is true.

This argument makes a strong case for type materialism.[5] To be sure, the case is only hypothetical – it stands or falls with the psychophysical

---

Metaphysical Controversy," in Philip Kitcher and Wesley C. Salmon (eds.), *Scientific Explanation* (Minneapolis: University of Minnesota Press, 1989), pp. 220–52)). There are also philosophers who think that the principle is clearly wrong (see, for example, Bas C. van Fraassen, *Laws and Symmetry* (Oxford: Oxford University Press, 1989, Part II).

This is not the place to mount a systematic defense of the best explanation principle. Suffice it to say that if the main objections were sound, they would discredit not only the best explanation principle but all other rules of ampliative inference as well. Thus, one should not embrace these objections unless one is also prepared to embrace a Humean skepticism about induction and science. (As I see it, with the exception of a couple of arguments that are closely related to certain strands in Hume's critique of induction, van Fraassen's objections presuppose interpretations of the best explanation principle that are extremely unsympathetic. I hope to comment on this set of objections elsewhere.)

5 Several other authors have noted that materialism can be defended by appealing to its explanatory power. Thus, as we will see, it is possible to construe a celebrated line of thought in one of Smart's papers as an argument of this sort. Further, although certain worries deter Lycan from accepting type materialism, Lycan states an argument that is similar to the one given earlier in his interesting paper on psychological laws. (See William G. Lycan, "Psychological Laws," *Philosophical Topics* 12 (1981), 9–38. He writes (p. 10) as follows: "What better way to explain a lawlike correlation between A's and B's than by supposing, in the absence of significant evidence to the contrary, that in fact A's *are* just B's.") Finally, in "Attribute-Identities in Microreductions" (*The Journal of Philosophy* LXIX (1972), 407–22), Robert L. Causey gives a general argument to the

correlation thesis. But it is a strong hypothetical case. If the correlation thesis can be defended empirically, and the philosophical objections to it can be met, then the argument will show decisively that type materialism is the correct answer to the mind–body problem.

It is clear, I think, that type materialism provides a good explanation of the psychophysical laws that are claimed to exist in the psychophysical correlation thesis. Suppose, for example, that conscious experiences of a certain kind ϕ turn out to be correlated with brain processes of kind ψ. Surely, if someone were to ask for an explanation of this correlation, it would be perfectly appropriate to respond by saying, "The correlation obtains because *being a conscious experience of type ϕ* is the very same thing as *being a brain process of type ψ*." (Compare: "Miss Lane, why does Clark Kent always turn up in the same places as Superman?" "Because, Jimmy, Clark *is* Superman.")

It is also clear that the explanations that type materialism provides compare favorably with the "explanations" of correlation laws that one finds in the writings of dualists. According to Leibniz, for example, the relationship between mind and body can only be explained by appealing to God's plan for the universe: It is like the relationship between two clocks that are designed in such a way that they remain in phase throughout their existence despite being causally isolated from one another. This account is inferior to the account provided by type materialism in a number of respects. For example, it is inferior in point of intelligibility. Although some philosophers hold that the concept of identity poses difficult problems, few if any deny that it is less problematical than the concept of God. Again, the explanation differs from the account provided by type materialism in that it raises more questions than it answers. If one were to explain psychophysical laws by appealing to the creative activity of God, one's account would inevitably lead to such questions as "Why did God want there to be events of two different kinds in the first place?" and "Why did God want events of the two kinds to be connected by the laws that actually exist?" On the other hand, there is no point to the question "Why is *being a conscious experience of type ϕ* identical with *being a brain process of type ψ*?" "*Being a conscious experience of type ϕ*" and "*being a brain process of*

---

effect that the plausibility of reductions derives from the explanatory power of propositions he calls "attribute-identity bridge laws." These propositions are identity statements.

type ψ" are names of properties. If a statement is constructed solely from the identity predicate and names, the statement holds in all possible worlds, and it is neither necessary nor possible to explain why the statement is true. (As Robert Causey says in a related context, such statements require justification but not explanation.[6])

It would be a mistake to look elsewhere among dualistic theories for better explanations. A dualistic "explanation" of a psychophysical law is usually little more than a euphemistic way of confessing that the law has the status of an unexplained primitive.

One encounters a somewhat different situation, however, when one considers the explanations of psychophysical laws that are offered by the double-aspect theory. Advocates of the theory need not accept the correlation thesis, but they are entitled to do so. Thus, there is a version of the double-aspect theory that is based on these claims: First, the correlation thesis is true; second, every event that is a token of some sensory property is identical with a token of the neural correlate of that property; and third, no sensory property is identical with any neural property. Like type materialism, this version of the double-aspect theory can explain all psychophysical laws claimed to exist in the correlation thesis without introducing metaphysical concepts that are highly problematic. When, for example, an advocate of the double-aspect theory is asked why conscious experiences of type ϕ accompany brain processes of type ψ, he or she can respond by saying that conscious experiences of type ϕ are *identical* with brain processes of type ψ. (Hereafter I will use the term "double-aspect theory" to refer to the particular version of the theory that is described in this paragraph.)

On the other hand, despite their similarity, the explanations provided by type materialism and the double-aspect theory are different in a key respect. To appreciate the difference, notice that both theories imply that there are a number of true generalizations of the following form:

> Every brain process of type ψ has the property *being a sensory event of type ϕ*. (1)

Type materialism can explain such generalizations, for substitution instances of (1) can be explained by substitution instances of "The property *being a brain process of type ψ* is identical with the property *being a sensory event of type ϕ*." But the double-aspect theory cannot give this

6 See Causey, ibid., pp. 413–14.

explanation. Nor does it have any other explanation to offer. Thus, the double-aspect theory replaces one set of facts with a new set of facts that are roughly similar to the first set, and it differs from type materialism in that it fails to explain the members of the new set.

III

Although, as I said at the outset, materialists have typically devoted more energy to criticizing dualists (and also one another) than to constructing positive arguments for materialism, it is widely held that the task of constructing a positive argument presents no serious difficulties. For it is widely held that it is possible in principle to justify materialism by an argument that is based on an appeal to simplicity. We find this view in, among other places, Smart's classic paper "Sensations and Brain Processes":

> [T]here is no conceivable experiment which could decide between materialism and epiphenomenalism. The latter issue is not like the average straight-out empirical issue in science, but like the issue between the nineteenth-century naturalist Philip Gosse and the orthodox geologists and paleontologists of his day. According to Gosse, the earth was created about 4000 B.C. exactly as described in Genesis, with twisted rock strata, "evidence" of erosion, and so forth, and all sorts of fossils, all in their appropriate strata, just as if the usual evolutionist story had been true. Clearly this theory is in a sense irrefutable: no evidence can possibly tell against it. Let us ignore the theological setting in which Philip Gosse's hypothesis had been placed, thus ruling out objections of a theological kind, such as "what a queer God who would go to such elaborate lengths to deceive us." Let us suppose that it is held that the universe just *began* in 4004 B.C. with the initial conditions just everywhere as they were in 4004 B.C., and in particular that our own planet began with sediment in the rivers, eroded cliffs, fossils in the rocks, and so on. No scientist would ever entertain this as a serious hypothesis, consistent though it is with all possible evidence. The hypothesis offends against the principles of parsimony and simplicity. There would be far too many brute and inexplicable facts. Why are pterodactyl bones just as they are? No explanation in terms of the evolution of pterodactyls from earlier forms of life would any longer be possible. We would have millions of facts about the world as it was in 4004 B.C. that just have to be accepted.
>
> The issue between the brain-process theory and epiphenomenalism seems to be of the above sort. (Assuming that a behavioristic reduction of introspective reports is not possible.) If it be agreed that there are no

cogent philosophical arguments which force us into accepting dualism, and if the brain-process theory and dualism are equally consistent with the facts, then the principles of parsimony and simplicity seem to me to decide overwhelmingly in favor of the brain-process theory. As I pointed out earlier, dualism involves a large number of irreducible psychophysical laws . . . of a queer sort, that just have to be taken on trust, and are just as difficult to swallow as the irreducible facts about the paleontology of the earth with which we are faced on Philip Gosse's theory.[7]

At first sight, it can seem that Smart is primarily concerned in this passage to justify materialism by appealing to its explanatory power. Thus, although he twice refers to parsimony and simplicity, it can seem that his main complaint against dualism is that it is committed to an unacceptably large number of "brute and *inexplicable* facts." This phrase, together with some of the surrounding material, suggests that Smart is more exercised by the explanatory impotence of dualism than by its complexity. However, there is a decisive reason for setting this interpretation aside, for in a later paper, Smart explicitly states that the argument in "Sensations and Brain Processes" is based on simplicity.[8]

Where *M* is any theory that is a form of materialism, it is no doubt possible to construct a simplicity argument that purports to show that *M* is to be preferred to dualism. However, I am primarily concerned here with type materialism, and I wish to focus on an argument that purports to show both that type materialism is superior to dualism and that it is superior to the double-aspect theory. This argument runs as follows:

> **First premise** (simplicity principle) If a theory T_1 is simpler than a competing theory T_2, then, all else being equal, there is a good and sufficient reason to prefer T_1 to T_2.
>
> **Second premise.** Type materialism is simpler than dualism and the double-aspect theory.
>
> **Conclusion.** There is a good and sufficient reason to prefer type materialism to dualism and the double-aspect theory.

Prima facie, at least, this argument has considerable appeal.

---

7 See J.J.C. Smart, "Sensations and Brain Processes," in David M. Rosenthal (Ed.), *Materialism and the Mind-Body Problem* (Englewood Cliffs: Prentice Hall, 1971), 53–66. The quoted passage occurs on pp. 65–66.

8 See J.J.C. Smart, "Ockham's Razor," in James H. Fetzer (ed.), *Principles of Philosophical Reasoning* (Totowa, NJ: Rowman and Allanheld, 1984), 118–28.

Unfortunately, the task of assessing the argument turns out to be rather complex. This is due in part to the fact that there are at least three distinguishable forms of simplicity.

First, there is *formal simplicity*. Formal simplicity is what we have in mind when we say that a given assumption is simpler than another because the former has a lower degree of logical complexity. It is also what we have in mind when we say that a given theory is simpler than another because the former has a smaller number of primitive assumptions. (Note that judgments of this second kind are intimately related to judgments of the first kind. A judgment of the second kind presupposes that the primitive assumptions of the theory that is said to be simpler are more or less equal to the primitive assumptions of the other theory in point of logical complexity. Without this rough equality, all theories would be equally simple, at least potentially, in point of number of primitive assumptions, for it is always possible to splice the assumptions of a theory together into a single proposition by forming their conjunction.)

Second, there is *ontological simplicity*. This is the form of simplicity that we have in mind when we say that one theory is simpler than another because the former posits a larger number of mutually irreducible categories of entities. (Some philosophers maintain that the ontological simplicity of a theory depends not only on the number of irreducible categories that the theory recognizes, but also on the number of entities in each of the categories. I have reservations about this stronger claim, and anyway, it is not especially relevant to the task of choosing between type materialism and its competitors. I will not be concerned with it here.)

Finally, there is a form that might be called *mathematical simplicity*. This is a property of theories that derives from the mathematical structure of the functions with which the theory is concerned, or, equivalently, from the curves that count as the graphical representations of these functions. Roughly speaking, the mathematical simplicity of a theory is a function of the smoothness of its associated curves. (Suppose we find by observation that a certain quantitative characteristic ϕ takes on the values $v_1, \ldots, v_n$ when a certain other characteristic ψ takes on the values $x_1, \ldots, x_n$. We want to choose a function that agrees with these findings, in the sense of yielding $v_1, \ldots, v_n$ when it is applied to $x_1, \ldots, x_n$, and that can reasonably be expected to yield correct values of ϕ when it is applied to new values of ψ. It is evident that the choice is not uniquely determined by our experimental findings: There are infinitely many functions that yield $v_1, \ldots, v_n$ when they are applied to $x_1, \ldots, x_n$ – that is, there are infinitely many curves that can be drawn through the points $(x_1, v_1), \ldots, (x_n, v_n)$. Any scientist would solve this problem by choosing the smoothest curve, and would describe this choice as the one that is required by considerations of simplicity.)

Now it is reasonably clear that we can set questions of mathematical simplicity aside in assessing the comparative merits of type materialism and its rivals. Type materialism is not associated in any interesting way with a distinctive set of functions or curves. Nor are its rivals. On the other hand, it seems to be possible to make meaningful comparisons between type materialism and its competitors with respect to both formal simplicity and ontological simplicity. So it seems that there are two ways of interpreting the foregoing argument. We need to take a closer look at both interpretations. We need to ask, "Does formal simplicity give us a reason to prefer type materialism to dualism and the double-aspect theory?" If so, what kind of reason does it give? (A cognitive reason? An aesthetic reason? A practical reason?) And is the reason strong? Further, does ontological simplicity give us a reason to prefer type materialism? If so, what kind of reason? And is the reason strong?

IV

Construed in accordance with the first interpretation, the simplicity argument looks like this:

> **First premise.** If a theory T_1 has a higher degree of formal simplicity than a competing theory T_2, then, all else being equal, there is a good and sufficient reason to prefer T_1 to T_2.

> **Second premise.** Type materialism has a higher degree of formal simplicity than dualism and the double-aspect theory.

> **Conclusion.** There is a good and sufficient reason to prefer type materialism to dualism and the double-aspect theory.

It is easier to assess the second premise than the first, so I will begin with it.

In order to facilitate comparisons, let us agree to view each of the three theories as a broadly inclusive system that incorporates all of the neurological information that is relevant to sensory states. That is to

29

say, let us suppose that each theory implies a set of purely neurological laws, a set of synchronic psychophysical laws, and a set of diachronic psychophysical laws. In addition, each of the theories offers its own distinctively philosophical account of the relationship between neural and sensory facts. Thus, type materialism asserts a set of statements that identify sensory state-types with neural state-types. Dualism makes a general claim to the effect that no sensory state-token is identical with any neural state-token (from which it follows, of course, that no sensory state-type is identical with any neural state-type). And the double-aspect theory puts forward a set of generalizations affirming the identity of sensory state-tokens with neural state-tokens (one generalization for each category or type of sensory state-token), and also a generalization to the effect that sensory state-types and neural state-types are numerically distinct.

Suppose now that we are concerned to organize each of these three systems into a formal theory. Suppose further that we are interested in finding an especially simple primitive basis for each of them. Which claims should we take as nonlogical axioms? In the case of type materialism it would suffice to select a set of axioms consisting in part of neurological laws and in part of statements affirming the identity of particular sensory state-types with particular neural state-types. We could then obtain the synchronic psychophysical laws and the dia-chronic psychophysical laws as theorems. In the case of dualism it would suffice to select a set consisting of three subsets: a subset composed of neurological laws, a subset composed of synchronic psy-chophysical laws (one for each of the type-identity statements in our axiomatization of type materialism), and a subset whose only member is the forementioned general statement denying the identity of sensory state-tokens with neural state-tokens. It would be possible to obtain the diachronic psychophysical laws as theorems. Finally, in the case of the double-aspect theory, we would again need to select a set consisting of three subsets: a subset composed of neurological laws, a subset com-posed of generalizations affirming the identity of sensory state-tokens with neural state-tokens (one for each of the synchronic psychophysical laws), and a subset whose sole member is the forementioned generali-zation concerning the nonidentity of sensory types with neural types. As in the case of type materialism, it would be possible to obtain both the synchronic psychophysical laws and the diachronic psychophysical laws as theorems.

As this account shows, type materialism requires fewer primitive assumptions than either of its rivals. And I see no reason for saying that it requires primitives with a higher degree of internal logical complexity. So it seems that type materialism comes out ahead of its rivals in point of formal simplicity. To be sure, the difference is small: The primitive basis for type materialism that I sketched has only one less primitive assumption than the other bases. But a small difference is still a difference, and any difference in formal simplicity is enough to show that the second premise is true.

What about the first premise? Is it really the case that formal simplicity is a good and sufficient reason for setting one theory aside in favor of another? In some cases the answer is clearly affirmative. Suppose that T_1 and T_2 are two substantive theories that have some claim on our assent but that are less deserving of our acceptance than the laws of logic. Suppose also that the primitive assumptions of T_1 are a proper subset of the primitive assumptions of T_2. And consider the conjunction law of the probability calculus. According to this law, the probability of the conjunction of the axioms of a theory is the same as the product of their individual probabilities. When this law is combined with our assumption about T_1 and T_2, we get the result that T_1 is more likely than T_2 to be true. (Assuming that the probability of a theory can be identified with the probability of the conjunction of its axioms, the conjunction law implies that we can obtain the probabilities of T_1 and T_2 by multiplying the individual probabilities of their constituent axioms. Suppose that r_1 and r_2 are the probabilities we are led to assign to T_1 and T_2, respectively. Suppose also that r_3 is the probability of the conjunction of the axioms that belong to T_2 but not to T_1. Because r_1, r_2, and r_3 are probabilities of substantive propositions that have some claim on our assent but that are less deserving of our acceptance than the laws of logic, they are all real numbers that are strictly greater than 0 and strictly smaller than 1. Further, since the axioms of T_1 are a subset of the axioms of T_2, the conjunction law implies that $r_2 = r_1 \times r_3$. It follows from these observations that r_2 is smaller than r_1.)

In a perfectly good sense of "reasonable," then, it is more reasonable to accept T_1 than to accept T_2. But this is only part of the story. If the primitive assumptions of T_1 are not a proper subset of the primitive assumptions of T_2, then even if the former primitives are fewer in number, it will not always be the case that T_1 is more probable than T_2.

Thus, suppose that T_1 is disjoint from T_2 and that each of the primitives of T_1 has a lower probability than any of the primitives of T_2. In a case of this sort, even if T_1 has fewer primitives than T_2, the conjunction law may still imply that T_2 should be preferred to T_1. The probability of a longer conjunction can be greater than the probability of a shorter one if the probabilities of its constituent statements are sufficiently high.

What about the case at hand? Can the conjunction law be used to show that type materialism is more probable than dualism? (I will set the double-aspect theory aside temporarily to simplify the exposition; but what I will say about the relationship between type materialism and dualism applies to the relationship between type materialism and the double-aspect theory as well.) The primitive assumptions of type materialism consist of neurological laws and statements affirming state-type identities. The primitive assumptions of dualism consist of neurological laws, synchronic psychophysical laws (one for each of the type-identity statements that type materialism takes as primitives), and the claim that sensory state-tokens are never identical with neural state-tokens. If we were in a position to say that each of the type-identity statements asserted by type materialism has the same probability as the corresponding psychophysical law, then, no matter what probability we assigned to dualism's negative claim about token-identities, type materialism would come out ahead. However, it seems that we have no right to assign the same probabilities to the type-identity statements and the synchronic psychophysical laws, for the former are stronger claims than the latter. (Each type-identity statement implies the corresponding psychophysical law, but the converse implications do not hold.) It seems that we should assign lower probabilities to the type-identity statements. But how much lower? If we wish to refrain from begging any questions, we will have to make assignments that are neutral between type materialism and dualism. Alas, this means that our assignments will have to be low indeed – so low as to prevent the probability of the conjunction of the type-identity statements from being higher than whatever probability we assign to the corresponding conjunction of statements from the dualist's theory (i.e., the conjunction consisting of the psychophysical laws and the claim that sensory state-tokens are distinct from neural state-tokens). The dualist will object to any assignment that violates this condition.

To summarize: In a case in which the primitive assumptions of one theory are a proper subset of the primitive assumptions of another, it does not matter what probabilities accrue to the individual components of the theories. No matter how one assigns probabilities to individual statements (short of assigning 0 or 1), it will be possible to show that the first theory is to be preferred to the other by an argument that is based on the conjunction law. But the situation is quite different in other cases. When there is no proper inclusion of primitive assumptions, everything depends on the probabilities of individual statements. Unfortunately, in the case at hand, it appears that there are no question-begging grounds for choosing a probability assignment that will make it possible for type materialists to exploit the conjunction law. No such assignment is forced upon us by a priori considerations or by empirical facts. Hence, any choice of an assignment of the sort in question would be challenged by the dualist.

Our task here is to determine whether it is possible to justify the first premise of the foregoing argument. We have considered the prospects of basing a justification on the notion of probability, and we have found them to be meager. We must now consider whether there is another way of approaching the problem.

For an explanation of the value of formal simplicity, one naturally turns to the work of Nelson Goodman. He writes:

> Science is systematization, and systematization is simplification. If discovery of a way of dispensing with one of Peano's postulates or a way of defining one of three primitives of a system in terms of the other two does not seem momentous, that is only by comparison with the enormous systematization already effected through deriving vastly many theorems or terms from so meager a basis. Some economies are indeed minor, but complete disregard for economy would imply a willingness to take all terms and statements as primitive, to waive all definition and proof, and so to forego all system. Without simplicity, there is no science.[9]

Here is another suggestive passage:

> Now why this insistence upon simplicity? Must not the righteous scientist rather aim at truth and only hope for simplicity? Efforts to simplify a theory are often thought to be merely for the sake of elegance; but actually simplification is the soul of science. Science consists not of collecting particular truths but of relating, defining, demonstrating, organizing – in short, of systematizing. And to systematize is to simplify; an integrated system is achieved just to the extent that everything can be reduced to a minimal apparatus of underived terms and statements – that

9 Nelson Goodman, "Science and Simplicity," in Goodman, *Problems and Projects* (Indianapolis: Bobbs-Merrill, 1972), 337–46. The quoted passage occurs on p. 338.

is, of undefined or primitive terms and postulates or axioms. Science is the search for the simplest applicable theory.[10]

I see two closely related but independent arguments in these passages. In the first one, Goodman points out that unless there is *some* formal simplicity, there is no distinction between the propositions we have assumed and the propositions we have proved. In the second, he points out that there is a strong positive correlation between formal simplicity and systematic organization, and that systematic organization is an important value, perhaps on a par with truth itself.

Although Goodman's arguments are insightful, I fear that they cannot provide much help in our present venture. As I presented them earlier, type materialism and dualism both have a fairly high degree of formal simplicity. Hence, there is no difficulty in either case in applying the distinction between what has been assumed and what has been proved. Moreover, as for systematic organization, the difference between them is marginal, consisting as it does of the fact that type materialism has one less primitive assumption than dualism. It would be ridiculous to try to settle a grand metaphysical dispute like that between type materialism and dualism by appealing to a difference as minute as this. (See Goodman's observation about the Peano postulates.)

In general, it seems that type materialism and dualism are sufficiently similar in point of formal simplicity that it is futile to attempt to use formal simplicity as the basis of an argument for type materialism. To be sure, small differences in formal simplicity can make for large differences in probability. (If the probability of a proposition is relatively low, it is possible to reduce the probability of a theory considerably by adding that proposition as a new assumption. Here a small reduction in formal simplicity is accompanied by a significant reduction in probability.) However, we have found reason to suspect that the relationship between type materialism and dualism is such as to prevent a probabilistic justification of the former from getting off the ground. And I know of no other important property of theories that satisfies the condition that large differences in the degrees of that property can accompany small differences in the cardinalities of sets of primitive assumptions. So it looks as though we need to move beyond formal

10 Nelson Goodman, "Uniformity and Simplicity," ibid., 347–54. The passage can be found on p. 351.

simplicity if we are to find an adequate version of the simplicity argument.

V

This brings us to the second version of the argument:

> **First premise.** If a theory T_1 has a higher degree of ontological simplicity than a competing theory T_2, then, all else being equal, there is a good and sufficient reason to prefer T_1 to T_2.
>
> **Second premise.** Type materialism has a higher degree of ontological simplicity than dualism and the double-aspect theory.
>
> **Conclusion.** There is a good and sufficient reason to prefer type materialism to dualism and the double-aspect theory.

After a word about the second premise, I will examine a couple of possible ways of justifying the first premise.

The second premise is in effect the conjunction of two independent claims. The idea underlying the first claim is that type materialism is simpler than dualism because it postulates fewer unreduced *events*. The idea underlying the second claim is that type materialism is simpler than the double-aspect theory because it postulates fewer unreduced *facts*. (The double-aspect theory asserts that there are things that exemplify both qualitative characteristics and physical characteristics, but because it denies that qualitative characteristics are identical with physical characteristics, it must reject the view that the fact that consists of something's exemplifying a qualitative characteristic is identical with any of the facts that consist of that thing's exemplifying a physical characteristic. So the double-aspect theory is committed to the existence of two irreducible categories of facts. Type materialism rejects this view.)

The second premise is eminently plausible. I think we should accept it.

The first premise is a version of a doctrine that seems to have been first promulgated by William of Ockham. Under the name "Ockham's Razor" the doctrine has long been a favorite of analytic philosophers. Thus, for example, Russell appealed to it in maintaining that because he had shown how to construct surrogates of the number systems within set theory, he was entitled to abstain from asserting the existence of numbers.[11]

---

11 See, for example, Bertrand Russell, *My Philosophical Development* (London: George Allen and Unwin, 1959), p. 71.

35

Although he may have held different views about the matter on other occasions, Russell was sometimes inclined to defend Ockham's Razor on the grounds that it contributes to epistemic *safety*. We find the following passage in *Mysticism and Logic*:

> Take again the case of cardinal numbers. Two equally numerous collections appear to have something in common: this something is supposed to be their cardinal number. But so long as the cardinal number is inferred from the collections, not constructed in terms of them, its existence must remain in doubt, unless in virtue of a metaphysical postulate ad hoc. By defining the cardinal number of a given collection as the class of all equally numerous collections, we avoid the necessity of this metaphysical postulate, and thereby remove a needless element of doubt from the philosophy of arithmetic.[12]

And in "The Philosophy of Logical Atomism" Russell wrote: "That is the advantage of Ockham's Razor, that it diminishes your risk of error."[13] Construed in the obvious way, these quotations indicate that Russell was inclined to justify the pursuit of ontological simplicity by appealing to probability of truth.

This idea works well enough in the cases with which Russell was primarily concerned – the case of numbers and the case of material objects. Take numbers. Suppose that it is true that set-theoretic surrogates of numbers can serve all of the mathematical purposes that are served by numbers themselves. Should we embrace numbers in addition to sets? Ockham's Razor indicates that the answer is negative. If he were asked to defend this answer, Russell could appeal to probability. Because we are committed to sets anyway, he could say, our total theory will make fewer existence claims if we decide to do without numbers than if we embrace them. Hence, the conjunction law of the probability calculus implies that the probability of our total theory will be higher if we decide to do without them. Or take material objects. Russell held that it is possible to construct surrogates of material objects out of sense data – surrogates that can serve all of the scientific purposes that material objects can serve. This belief is almost certainly false, but let us suppose for a moment that it is correct. Should we embrace material objects in addition to sense data? Once again, Ock-

---

12 See Bertrand Russell, *Mysticism and Logic* (New York: Doubleday, 1957), p. 156.
13 See Bertrand Russell, "The Philosophy of Logical Atomism," in R.C. Marsh (ed.), *Logic and Knowledge* (New York: G.P. Putnam's Sons, 1956), 177–281. The quotation comes from p. 280.

ham's Razor calls for a negative answer. And once again it is possible to defend a negative answer by appealing to the probability of truth. Because our total theory will make fewer existence claims if we decide to do without material objects, the conjunction law implies that we should refrain from embracing them.

We can see a common pattern in these cases. In each case there are two theories, T_1 and T_2, where T_2 contains all of the assertions of T_1, and a number of others besides, including some existential assertions. The question arises: Should we drop T_2 while continuing to use T_1? In both cases there are two considerations that favor a positive answer. First, we have no need of the additional assertions that are made by T_2; it is possible to get by with the assertions of T_1. Second, we can increase our epistemic safety by jettisoning T_2; for the conjunction law is applicable, and it implies that the probability of T_2 is lower than the probability of T_1.

We have a schema here that can be applied in other cases. It seems that whenever we have a pair of theories that fulfill the conditions on T_1 and T_2, we are entitled to amputate the assertions that belong to T_2 but not to T_1. (Note that the schema can be generalized: our right to perform this sort of amputation is not limited to existential assertions, or even to cases in which existential assertions are involved.)

Here, however, we must take note of an important restriction. The assertions of T_1 must be a proper subset of the assertions of T_2. If T_1 contains assertions that are not components of T_2, then, even if T_1 and T_2 overlap to a considerable degree, it will not be possible to justify a preference for T_1 by a straightforward application of the conjunction law. For the probabilities of the components of T_1 that do not belong to T_2 might very well lower the probability of T_1 to the same degree or to an even greater degree than the probability of T_2 is lowered by the probabilities of the components of T_2 that are not components of T_1.

This is in fact the situation we encounter when we turn from comparing theories (1) and (2):

(1) Set theory

(2) The theory consisting of set theory, number theory, and the proposition that numbers have an independent existence

with the task of comparing (2) with (3):

(3) The theory consisting of set theory, number theory, and the proposition that numbers are reducible to sets.

(2) makes an existential claim that (3) refrains from making (namely, the claim that there are entities in addition to sets). However, even though (3) must for this reason be said to have a greater amount of ontological

simplicity than (2), it is far from clear that the probability of (3) is higher. This can be seen by comparing (3) with (1). Whereas (1) cautiously remains neutral on the question of the independent existence of numbers, (3) in effect denies that numbers exist as independent entities. This shows a great deal of epistemic daring – so much that it seems natural to say that (3) takes as large an epistemic risk as (2).

In order to establish that (3) has a higher probability than (2) it would be necessary to give an independent argument – that is, an argument that is not based on Ockham's Razor – to show that there is something uniquely problematical about the idea that numbers have an independent existence, or to give an independent argument to show that assertions of irreducibility are generally in a high-risk category, in the sense that they are more likely to be false than assertions of other kinds. An argument of either of these sorts would involve a lot more than an appeal to the conjunction law.

How do things stand in the case of sensations? Can we give a Russellian argument to show that type materialism is to be preferred to dualism? (Once again I set the double-aspect theory aside in the interests of brevity.) Can we say that type materialism and dualism satisfy the conditions on T_1 and T_2 in the schema we noticed a bit earlier? Obviously not. Rather, the relationship between dualism and type materialism is like the relationship between (2) and (3). It is true that dualism makes two existential claims that are foreign to type materialism – it asserts the existence of nonphysical characteristics, and it asserts the existence of nonphysical events. In doing so it takes an epistemic risk. However, type materialism takes a risk as well, for it makes some substantive claims of its own. Specifically, it puts forward claims that challenge the existential assertions of dualism: It denies that sensory characteristics are nonphysical, and also that sensory events are nonphysical. Is the risk that dualism incurs any greater than the risk that is associated with type materialism? I doubt it. To show that it is greater, it would be necessary to show that there is something uniquely problematical about the existence of nonphysical characteristics or nonphysical events, or to show that assertions of irreducibility are generally in a high-risk category. I despair of finding an argument of either of these kinds. (Moreover, an argument of the first kind would not count, strictly speaking, as an appeal to ontological simplicity. The real work would not be done by the observation that type materialism commits us to fewer kinds of entities than dualism, but rather by the claim that dualism commits us to entities of questionable virtue.)

Russell's idea, as I have interpreted it, was to give a probabilistic justification for the use of Ockham's Razor. This idea works brilliantly in some cases, but seems not to work in the case that is before us here.[14, 15] As I see it, if we are to find a rationale for using Ockham's Razor, we must look in a different direction. Instead of looking for a

14 Here I can imagine someone arguing as follows: "It is possible to give a probabilistic justification of a restricted version of Ockham's Razor that is entirely independent of Russell's justification. Thus, it is apparent that there is only a finite number of types of concrete objects and events that have instances in the actual world. ('Type' is being used here as an equivalent of 'universal.') Further, it is plausible to say that there are infinitely many types of concrete objects and events that have no actual instances. (For surely it is correct to say that there are infinitely many types that would have had instances if cosmogony or evolution had taken a different course.) Hence, the set of types that have instances is only a tiny fragment of the set of all types. Suppose now that we impose a probability measure on the set of all types. Given that the set of types with actual instances is only a tiny fragment of the set of all types, it must be true that if someone were to choose a type randomly from the latter set, the probability of his picking a type with actual instances would be vanishingly small. But then we must conclude that where E is any assertion that affirms the existence of an instance of some type, E has an a priori probability that is extremely low."

Although this argument is suggestive and moderately convincing, I question its relevance. It would be highly relevant if we were comparing existential assertions with their denials (provided the assertions were concerned with types of concrete objects or events). But we aren't. Instead we are comparing assertions of the form "There exist A's and B's and the A's are not reducible to the B's" with assertions of the form "There exist A's and B's and the A's are reducible to the B's." We cannot draw any conclusions from the foregoing argument about the probabilities of statements of the latter two forms. Nor, as far as I can see, is there any related argument which provides support for such conclusions.

15 Thus far we have been concerned exclusively with the question of whether it is possible to give an a priori justification for a suitable version of Ockham's Razor. But it might be suggested that it is possible to come up with an a posteriori justification for a suitable version (by arguing inductively that as a matter of empirical fact, simple theories are quite likely to be true).

I do not wish to deny that this approach could provide us with an adequate justification of a principle of simplicity of some kind, but I doubt very much that it could deliver a version of Ockham's Razor that is strong enough to establish type materialism. This is because a wide range of the types that are recognized in the sciences appear to resist reduction. There is a well-known argument that this is true of many of the types that are recognized in the social sciences in Jerry A. Fodor's *The Language of Thought* (Cambridge, MA: Harvard University Press, 1975). This argument is quite convincing. And there are many other arguments of the same sort – for example, there are convincing arguments that such secondary qualities as color and temperature are not reducible. (See Clyde L. Hardin, *Color for Philosophers* (Indianapolis: Hackett Publishing Company, 1988), and Mark Wilson, "What is this Thing Called 'Pain'? – The Philosophy of Science Behind the Contemporary Debate," *Pacific Philosophical Quarterly* 66 (1985), 227–67.) In view of considerations of this sort, it seems unreasonable to think that there could be a strong inductive argument for a version of Ockham's Razor that implied that theories that include type-reducibility claims are quite likely to be true.

cognitive justification, we need to explore the possibility that the pursuit of ontological simplicity can be justified by aesthetic considerations.

Theories with comparatively few existential commitments tend to appeal to our aesthetic sensibilities. This can be seen by reflecting on type materialism itself. Type materialism has no tendency to deny or to deemphasize the diversity of the constituents of the universe, but it implies that there is a fundamental homogeneity at the deepest level. It also implies that the universe has a high degree of cohesiveness. It tells us that the constituents of the universe are connected by a comparatively small set of forces. In other words, type materialism represents the world as having a kind of homogeneity that is compatible with complexity and diversity, and as being highly unified and integrated. These are qualities that we care about, qualities that we find intrinsically valuable. It seems reasonable to say that, all else being equal, if a theory represents the universe as having these qualities, there is a reason to prefer that theory to its competitors.

Type materialism represents the universe as uniform and unified, and dualism represents it as bifurcated and syncretic. So there is an aesthetic argument for type materialism. Is it a strong argument? Yes, but we must distinguish between strength and generality of appeal. Some of us have vivid aesthetic intuitions that count in favor of ontological simplicity. Those in this category will be inclined to say that the argument makes a strong case for type materialism. However, it appears that aesthetic intuitions are highly diverse. This is clearly true of intuitions concerning the comparative merits of works of art, and it may also be true of intuitions concerning the value of ontological simplicity.

It seems, then, that my claim for the simplicity argument must be modest. I must not maintain that it can be used to establish that type materialism is probable, nor that it can be used to convert all rational beings to type materialism. Rather, I can claim only that the argument makes a case that will be found persuasive by people whose aesthetic intuitions cause them to attach importance to ontological simplicity. It is, of course, my hope that the reader will find on reflection that he or she belongs to this group.[16]

16 At this point, a reader of Elliott Sober's important book on simplicity might suggest that we should look for inspiration there. (See Sober, *Simplicity* (Oxford: Oxford University Press, 1975).)

VI

Thus far we have found two ways of arguing for the superiority of type materialism – the best explanation argument, and the version of the simplicity argument that we have just been considering. Is there a third way?

In addition to maintaining that dualism is in violation of the requirements of simplicity, the early materialists charged that dualism fails to provide a satisfactory account of the causal roles of sensations. Thus, the materialists took it as a nonnegotiable assumption that there is causal interaction between sensations and brain processes. They went on to maintain that dualism lacks the resources to explain either *how* brain processes produce sensations or *how* sensations can influence the brain.

Arguments of this sort are not completely without merit. In my judgment, however, they do not add very much to the arguments we have already considered.

Sober maintains that all simplicity judgments derive from a single notion of simplicity: In his account, mathematical simplicity, formal simplicity, and ontological simplicity are branches of a single tree. He explains a technical concept that he describes as a concept of information, and he then argues that the simplicity of a hypothesis is always directly proportional to the amount of information that the hypothesis contains. Once this argument is in hand, he goes on to identify simplicity with information content.

Much of what Sober says is illuminating. However, in my judgment, there is only one sense of "information" in which it is both true and important that type materialism is more informative than dualism, and Sober's theory does not capture this sense. In the sense in question, "informative" comes to the same thing as "having a significant amount of explanatory power." As I see it, then, the only worthwhile argument for type materialism that is based on a notion of information is an argument that we have already considered – namely, the best explanation argument.

Further, I have some worries about the content of Sober's theory. For one thing, I think it is a mistake to attempt to give a uniform account of the various forms of simplicity. (The forms can diverge. For example, ZF set theory has a higher degree of ontological simplicity than NGB set theory (ZF posits one category of entities and NGB posits two), but it has a much lower degree of formal simplicity (ZF has an infinite number of axioms and NGB has a finite number).) In addition, certain of Sober's claims concerning the comparative simplicity of particular kinds of hypotheses conflict with our intuitions. (For an insightful discussion of this point, see Richard W. Miller, *Fact and Method* (Princeton: Princeton University Press, 1987) pp. 254–58.) In general, Sober's theory seems to be more in keeping with our intuitions when it is taken as an account of the power of a hypothesis to simplify the task of answering a question than when it is as an account of the simplicity of a hypothesis.

My reasons for not discussing certain theories of simplicity that are related to Sober's theory, such as Sir Karl Popper's theory, are connected with these worries about Sober's position.

41

It is of course true that dualism fails to explain how sensations interact with brain states. It simply takes their interaction as primitive. But there is no intrinsic absurdity here. There is nothing wrong with denying that a certain form of causal interaction can be explained in terms of factors that operate at some deeper level. Indeed, physics itself countenances a range of primitive causal interactions – it *must* do so if it is to avoid postulating an infinite number of levels of explanation.

This is not to deny that it is possible to argue for type materialism by appealing to causal roles. One can do so as follows:

> In proposing a reduction of sensations to brain states, type materialism in effect proposes a reduction of psychophysical causal relations to neural causal relations; for the former reduction enables us to deduce psycho-physical causal laws from the laws of neurophysiology. Unlike dualism, therefore, type materialism is able to explain the causal roles of sensa-tions. But, according to the best explanation principle, we should prefer type materialism to dualism.

This argument makes a pretty strong case for type materialism, but it does not add significantly to the case we have already constructed. We already have an argument that is based on the best explanation principle. What we are looking for is an argument with a different foundation.

In general, materialist arguments that involve appeals to the causal roles of sensations tend to fall into two categories. Some leave dualists a lot of room in which to maneuver. Others are more conclusive; but the members of this second category generally involve appeals to simplicity or to explanatory power, and it would therefore be wrong to think of them as fundamentally different from the arguments we have already considered.

Before concluding, I will comment briefly on a line of thought that is quite different than the arguments we have considered thus far.

It seems that there is broad inductive support for the thesis that all concrete particulars – all natural objects and natural events – are composed of physical particulars, in the sense of being made of objects and/or events that are ultimately physical in nature. This thesis has frequently been noted in the literature on reduction. We find it, for example, in two classic papers on physicalism by Hellman and Thompson.[17] Calling it the *principle of physical exhaustion*, Hellman and Thompson formulate the thesis as follows:

17 See Geoffrey Hellman and Frank W. Thompson, "Physicalism: Ontology, Determina-tion, and Reduction," *The Journal of Philosophy* LXXII (1975), 551–64, and "Physicalist Materialiam," *Nous* 11 (1977), 309–45.

> Our ontology includes at the very least all concrete referents of the terms of basic physical theory. In addition it includes every part or sum of parts of the entities initially accepted. Finally, our mathematical-physical ontology includes every object occurring at any level of an ordinary set-theoretic hierarchy taking as urelements the null set and the entities already recognized. The [Principle of Physical Exhaustion] holds that the universe so delineated embraces everything there is.[18]

It is plausible to say that this principle has received strong support from the march of science during the last two centuries, and that we are therefore fully entitled today to claim to have a posteriori knowledge of its truth.

Further, it seems entirely appropriate to count sensations as natural events: They are located in time and, by most accounts, in space (though dualistic doctrines often deny that they have "definite" locations in space), and they depend nomologically for their existence on events that are paradigmatically natural (namely, brain processes). Hence, it seems entirely appropriate to think that sensations fall under generalizations that apply to all natural objects and events, and in particular, to think that they fall under the principle of physical exhaustion. But then dualism must be false.

This is a persuasive argument. However, it is of limited value in the present context, for it is purely negative. It tells us that dualism is false, but, as it stands, it has no tendency to show that type materialism is to be preferred to dualism. Moreover, it is limited in scope: As it stands, it has no tendency to show that the double-aspect theory is false.

Can it be expanded to an argument that supports type materialism? Or to an argument that counts against the double-aspect theory? Probably not. To be in a position to extend it in either of these directions, we would have to be able to supplement the principle of physical exhaustion with a principle to the effect that the state-types that are recognized in the special sciences tend to be reducible to the state-types that are postulated by more basic sciences. And, as I urged in note 15, it seems that the prospects of our being able to establish such a principle are extremely dim.

So, in addition to the reasons given earlier, there is an a posteriori reason to doubt that dualism is true. But it seems that there is no a posteriori reason – no strong reason – for embracing type materialism or for rejecting the double-aspect theory.

18 See Hellman and Thompson, "Physicalist Materialism," p. 310.

3

The failings of functionalism

We are concerned here to understand the ultimate metaphysical nature of both sensations and qualitative characteristics. Apart from the behaviorist doctrine that sensations can be reduced to congeries of behavioral dispositions, and the eliminativist thesis that the existence of sensations is in some sense fictional, both of which seem to me to be wildly implausible, there are just four views that one can take of these matters – type materialism, dualism, the double-aspect theory, and functionalism. We have reached the conclusion that, under certain assumptions, type materialism is to be preferred to dualism and the double-aspect theory. It is time now to look at functionalism.

Functionalism is broadly relevant to most of the main concerns of the philosophy of mind. It gives us a unified perspective from which to view sensations, emotions, the will, the nature of the self, and propositional attitudes (belief, desire, intention, and the other mental states that seem to involve relations to propositions). Here I wish to focus on those aspects of functionalism that are concerned with the sensory realm. Because of this, my exposition of functionalist doctrines will sidestep some technical questions that would have to be faced if we were considering the functionalist account of propositional attitudes. Further, my criticisms of functionalism will be directed only against its claims about sensations. They are not intended to call other functionalist doctrines into question. Indeed, even though I am convinced that the functionalist theory of sensations is hopelessly misguided, I think it likely that certain other parts of functionalism are sound.

My grasp of the content of functionalism and my conception of its flaws have been shaped to a large degree by a paper by Ned Block (cited in note 10), and by Block's inspiring lectures at the 1981 Summer Institute on Psychology and the Philosophy of Mind. I have also been helped substantially by conversations with Richard Lee, Lowell Nissen, and Sydney Shoemaker.

I

Functionalism was originally inspired and continues to be informed by a set of perceptions concerning the distribution of mental states.[1] According to functionalists, we have vivid intuitions to the effect that mental states are distributed across an extremely broad spectrum of biological species. It is claimed that we are strongly inclined to ascribe mental states to bats, octopi, and lobsters, and even to snakes, spiders, and crickets. Further, functionalists maintain that we are strongly inclined to ascribe mental states to certain nonbiological beings – in particular, to certain of the androids that we encounter in the realms of science fiction. We feel sure, it is said, that C3PO and R2D2 enjoy beliefs and desires, that they are subject to emotions, and that they are capable of having sensations of various kinds. Perhaps we are not entirely sure that, for example, C3PO can experience pain, but that is only because he is a less-than-perfect replica of ourselves. If an android had a nervous system that was fully isomorphic to a human nervous system – in the sense that there was a one-to-one structure-preserving correspondence between the artificial neurons of the android and the real neurons of a human brain – we would be entirely confident that the android had the capacity to feel pain.

According to functionalists, then, we are committed to ascribing mental states to beings who are composed of the same sort of matter as ourselves, but whose brains differ from ours in neuroanatomical structure. And we are also committed to ascribing mental states to beings whose brains may be structurally similar to ours, but who differ from us in material composition. Evidently, if these perceptions are correct, it would be a mistake to suppose that psychological characteristics are universally correlated with neural state-types of any sort. (Here and elsewhere, I use "state type" to stand for characteristics whose instances are all similar in their intrinsic natures – that is, I use it as an equivalent of "universal.") Indeed, if the perceptions are correct, it would be a mistake to suppose that psychological characteristics are universally correlated wtih physical state-types of any kind (where a state-type counts as physical if it is definable either in terms of the

---

1 Hilary Putnam, the father of functionalism, was the first to articulate these perceptions. See the papers on Philosophy of Mind collected in his *Mind, Language and Reality* (Cambridge: Cambridge University Press, 1975).

vocabulary of biology or in terms of the vocabulary of some more "basic" science such as chemistry or physics). A fortiori, it would be a mistake to suppose that there can be a physicalist reduction of psychological characteristics.

If functionalism denies that pain can be reduced to a physical state-type, what positive account of pain does it offer? What does it tell us about the nature of pain? According to functionalism, if an internal event counts as a pain, it does so because it exemplifies a state-type that plays a certain *causal* or *functional role* in the being in whom it occurs. What role? Functionalists differ in their responses to this question. However, it is not atypical for functionalists to say something like this: Where λ is a state-type, λ plays the role of pain in beings of type β just in case (1) events that exemplify λ tend to be caused by events that are actually or potentially harmful to beings of type β (that is, by events that actually cause bodily damage or threaten to cause such damage), (2) events that exemplify λ tend to cause withdrawal in beings of type β from harmful stimuli and nursing of damaged bodily parts, and (3) events that exemplify λ also tend to cause certain other types of internal event in beings of type β, such as feelings of distress and thoughts about ways of obtaining relief. Functionalists who favor this view of the functional role of pain maintain that any state-type that plays this role (in beings of some determinate kind) is a form of pain. Moreover, because functionalists also maintain that different state-types play the role in beings of different kinds, they are led to claim that pain itself – the property that is exemplified by all concrete events that count as cases of pain – is best analyzed as the property of being a concrete event x such that x exemplifies a state-type that plays the role in the members of some category of beings. In other words, where χ is the role in question, functionalists are led to claim that pain is identical with the property ϕ such that, necessarily, a concrete event x exemplifies ϕ if and only if there is some state-type such that (1) this state-type is exemplified by x, and (2) the state-type plays role χ in the being in whom x occurred (and in other beings of the same kind).

This view about pain is typical of functionalist doctrines generally. Functionalists maintain that psychological properties are always correlated uniquely with functional roles, and that each such property can be identified with the property of being a state-token x such that x exemplifies a state-type that plays the associated role in the being in whom x occurred (and in similar beings).

It will be useful to say more here about the key notions in this account.

There is a familiar distinction between properties that are first order and properties that are second order: First-order properties are exemplified by individual substances and concrete events, and second-order properties are exemplified by other properties – in particular, by first-order properties. Where χ is a second-order property, χ counts as a *functional role* if and only if it satisfies this condition: If λ is a first-order property, λ exemplifies χ if and only if (1) λ is a state-type that can be exemplified by internal state-tokens of some system S, and (2) λ is linked by causal (or probabilistic) laws to other properties of internal state-tokens of S, to properties of outputs of S, to properties of inputs of S, and/or to properties of distal stimuli to which S can be seen to be sensitive. Further, if a first-order property exemplifies a functional role with respect to some system S, the property is said to *play* that role in S. Equivalently, the property is said to *occupy* the role in S, and to *realize* the role in S.[2]

Where χ is a functional role, there is a unique property (a *functional property*) that is associated with χ – namely, the property of being a token of some state-type that realizes χ in the being in whom the token occurred (and in similar beings). Because this correspondence between functional roles and functional properties is one-to-one, and because functionalists maintain that the correspondence between psychological properties and functional roles is one-to-one, functionalists are committed to the view that every psychological property corresponds uniquely to a functional property. Building on this commitment, they affirm the central thesis of functionalism: Every psychological property is identical with a functional property.[3] (It is necessary to identify psychological properties with functional properties rather than func-

2 This way of looking at functional roles seems to have first been made fully explicit by Brian Loar. See his *Mind and Meaning* (Cambridge: Cambridge University Press, 1981), Chapter 3.
3 There are philosophers who are sometimes called "functionalists" whose positions are not captured by this formula. (Perhaps the most influential figure of this sort is David Lewis. See his "Mad Pain and Martian Pain" in Ned Block (ed.), *Readings in Philosophy of Psychology*, Vol. I (Cambridge, MA: Harvard University Press, 1980), 217–22.) I wish to claim only that the formula captures the views of typical functionalists.

  Although my exposition of functionalism is intended to apply only to the views that belong to the mainstream, I raise several objections to functionalism that count against deviant versions as well as typical ones.

tional roles because psychological properties and functional properties are both first-order. It would be absurd to identify properties that belong to different logical types.)

What, according to functionalism, is the relationship between the mental and the physical? The answer is complex. As a matter of sociological fact, most functionalists hold that every token of a psychological property is ultimately physical in nature, in the sense of being identical with something that is a token of a physical property. By the same token, where χ is the functional role that corresponds to a psychological property, and A is the set of state-types that realize χ, most functionalists maintain that the members of A must be physical properties. Thus, functionalists tend to favor a worldview that is markedly physicalist. However, there is nothing about functionalism that requires its adherents to opt for a physicalist ontology; it is in principle possible for a functionalist to endorse a version of dualism. For example, a functionalist could hold that the state-type that occupies the functional role of pain in human beings is a Cartesian property (that is, a property of concrete entities that entails that the entities that exemplify it are nonphysical). One might decide to reject this view. But if one does decide to reject it, it will have to be on grounds that are independent of functionalism. In its purest form, functionalism is the doctrine that psychological properties are identical with functional properties. Period. It makes no claims about the nature of properties that realize functional roles.

What are the reasons for accepting functionalism? The most important reason derives from the following correlation thesis: Where ψ is any psychological characteristic, there exists a functional property ϕ such that (1) instances of ψ are always instances of ϕ, and (2) instances of ϕ are always instances of ψ. Functionalists maintain that this thesis is correct. Clearly, if they are right, we must seek an explanation of the correlations that it claims to exist. And functionalism provides an explanation. Moreover, it provides the best explanation. How could one improve on the proposition that the correlations occur because psychological characteristics are identical with functional properties? This explanation deserves to receive the highest possible marks for clarity, simplicity, and completeness. Hence, by the best explanation principle, we have a good and sufficient reason for thinking that functionalism is true.

Second, it is sometimes maintained that functionalism can be seen to be true by reflecting on the meanings of terms in our psychological vocabulary. We find a line of thought of this sort in Smart's famous defense of an early form of functionalism. Although he regarded token-identity statements like "my current yellowish-orange after-image = the electro-chemical processes in my *B* fibers" as true, it was obvious to Smart that they are fully synthetic, and he took this to show that the meanings of sensation terms are equally compatible with dualism and materialism. Thus, while he thought that such terms must have complex meanings that could be brought to the fore by philosophical analysis, he also thought that any such analysis must be metaphysically neutral. After reflection he came to the conclusion that meanings of terms for sensations can be analyzed by descriptions that pick out internal states by specifying their relations to external phenomena. For example, he maintained that when "a person says: 'I see a yellowish-orange after-image,' he is saying something like this: '*There is something going on which is like what is going on when* I have my eyes open, am awake, and there is an orange illuminated in good light in front of me, that is, when I really see an orange'."[4] Smart went on as follows:

> Notice that the italicized words, namely "there is something going on which is like what is going on when," are all quasilogical or topic neutral words. This explains why the ancient Greek peasant's reports about his sensations can be neutral between dualistic metaphysics and my materialistic metaphysics. It explains how sensations can be brain-processes and yet how a man who reports them need know nothing about brain processes.[5]

What we have here is a semantic defense of a quasifunctionalist doctrine. Thus, it seems appropriate to characterize these two passages as follows: The first passage puts forward a view that entails that "yellowish-orange after-image" stands for a quasi-functional property; and the second passage urges that this view be accepted because it provides the best explanation of some important semantic facts. (I say that the view entails that "yellowish-orange after-image" stands for a *quasi*functional property because the property in question is one that internal phenomena have solely by virtue of their (indirect) relations to inputs; an event could have this property even if it had no tendency to cause memories or beliefs or any other internal phenomena, and even if

---

4 See J.J.C. Smart, "Sensations and Brain Processes" in David Rosenthal (ed.), *Materialism and the Mind–Body Problem* (Englewood Cliffs: Prentice Hall, 1971), 53–66. The quoted passage occurs on p. 61.
5 Smart, ibid., p. 51.

it had no tendency to cause outputs. Paradigmatic functional properties are more complex.)

There is also a third argument for functionalism – an argument that is due to Sydney Shoemaker. According to this line of thought, if we reject the functionalist account of qualitative characteristics, we will have no way of resisting a skeptic who maintains that we cannot be said to have knowledge of our qualitative states. Thus, Shoemaker in effect defends functionalism by maintaining that the cost of rejecting it is prohibitively high.

This third argument is eminently worthy of our attention, but I will not say any more about it here. It is best to defer consideration of it until we have taken a closer look at the nature of introspective awareness of sensations. We will return to it in Chapter 6.

II

Our picture of functionalism is still incomplete. To obtain a complete picture, we must take note of the fact that there is a systematic correspondence between classes of functional properties and psychological theories – a correspondence that can be expressed by saying that every psychological theory determines a class of functional properties. Once we have a feeling for this correspondence, we will be in a position to appreciate the functionalist strategy for obtaining accounts of the distinctive natures of individual psychological properties, and we will also be able to grasp the differences between the two main varieties of functionalism.

Now, a psychological theory can be represented by a single sentence, for we can always combine the basic laws of a theory into one law by taking their conjunction. Suppose that $P(T_1, \ldots, T_n, I_1, \ldots, I_j, O_1, \ldots, O_p)$ is a sentence that represents a psychological theory, that $T_1, \ldots, T_n$ is a list of the terms of the theory that stand for internal state-types, that $I_1, \ldots, I_j$ is a list of the terms that stand for types of inputs, and that $O_1, \ldots, O_p$ is a list of the terms that stand for types of outputs.[6] In addition, suppose that $P(X_1, \ldots, X_n, I_1, \ldots, I_j,$

---

6 Here I am assuming that the T_i's, the I_i's, and the O_i's are all singular terms. (I make this assumption because it allows me to formalize the definitions given in ensuing paragraphs in first-order logic.)

It is a bit unusual for a theory to pick out properties by singular terms rather than predicates. It is, however, possible to focus on theories of this kind without sacrificing generality, for it is always possible to translate a theory that is based on a vocabulary of

50

$O_1, \ldots, O_p$) is the result of replacing $T_1, \ldots, T_n$ with property variables (i.e., variables that range over properties rather than concrete objects or events).

This second sentence does not refer to any internal state-types in particular, but rather expresses a condition that is satisfied by some internal state-types and not by others. The condition in question can be characterized by saying what is involved in satisfying it. Specifically, it can be characterized as follows: Where $<\phi_1, \ldots, \phi_n>$ is a sequence of n internal state-types, $<\phi_1, \ldots, \phi_n>$ satisfies the condition expressed by $P(X_1, \ldots, X_n, I_1, \ldots, I_j, O_1, \ldots, O_p)$ if and only if the ϕ_i's stand in certain relations (namely, the causal and probabilistic relations expressed by the laws of the original theory) to one another and to the inputs $I_1, \ldots, I_j$ and the outputs $O_1, \ldots, O_p$.

Let us now consider (1):

> There exist state-types $X_1, \ldots, X_n$ such that (a) $P(X_1, \ldots, X_n, I_1, \ldots, I_j, O_1, \ldots, O_p)$, and (b) y exemplifies X_1.   (1)

The variable "y" in clause (b) is to be thought of as ranging over concrete entities – tokens of the internal states of the beings with which $P(T_1, \ldots, T_n, I_1, \ldots, I_j, O_1, \ldots, O_p)$ is concerned. Accordingly, (1) expresses a property of such tokens. Specifically, it expresses the property that is exemplified by a concrete state-token y if and only if y exemplifies the state-type that is the first member of some sequence of state-types that satisfies the condition expressed by $P(X_1, \ldots, X_n, I_1, \ldots, I_j, O_1, \ldots, O_p)$. In other words, it expresses the property of exemplifying some state-type or other that is the first member of a sequence of state-types that satisfies this condition.

(1) does not single out any sequence of state-types in particular, but still, it manages to express a perfectly determinate property. This can

---

seem miraculous, but in fact it is an instance of a phenomenon that is rather prosaic. Thus, compare (1) with the following sentence:

There exists a person z such that y is the mother of z.

This expresses the property of being the mother of some person or other (the property of being a mother, for short). Similarly, (1) expresses the property of being an internal state-token that exemplifies some state-type that is the first member of a sequence of state-types such that the members of this sequence satisfy the condition expressed by $P(X_1, \ldots, X_n, I_1, \ldots, I_j, O_1, \ldots, O_p)$. In both cases the property that is expressed is fully determinate, but we use a "topic-neutral" expression (consisting of an existence condition and one or more variables) in picking that property out.

The property expressed by (1) meets the conditions in the foregoing definition of the notion of a functional property.

Suppose now that we prefix the operator "being a state-token y such that" to (1). This gives us (2):

> Being a state-token y such that there exist state-types $X_1, \ldots, X_n$ such that (a) $P(X_1, \ldots, X_n, I_1, \ldots, I_j, O_1, \ldots, O_p)$, and (b) y exemplifies X_1. (2)

(2) is a singular term that refers to the property that is expressed by (1).

There are n descriptions associated with $P(T_1, \ldots, T_n, I_1, \ldots, I_j, O_1, \ldots, O_p)$ that have the same form as (2), one for each of the n T_i's. Let us agree to call them all *Ramsey functional descriptions*. (They are named for F.P. Ramsey, the logician who discovered the techniques that we are exploiting here.) Further, for each term T_i, let us agree to say that (3):

> being a state-token y such that there exist state-types $X_1, \ldots, X_n$ such that (a) $P(X_1, \ldots, X_n, I_i, \ldots, I_j, O_1, \ldots, O_p)$, and (b) y exemplifies X_i (3)

is the *Ramsey functional description (associated with $P(T_1, \ldots, T_n, I_1, \ldots, I_j, O_1, \ldots, O_p)$) that corresponds to T_i*. Let us also agree to say that the property named by (3) is the *ith Ramsey functional correlate of* $P(T_1, \ldots, T_n, I_1, \ldots, I_j, O_1, \ldots, O_p)$. Finally, a theory may be said to *determine* a set of functional properties if the members of the set are the Ramsey functional correlates for the theory.[7]

---

7 Although these definitions are perfectly standard, they mask some technical problems that take on considerable importance when one turns from the functionalist doctrine of qualia and takes up the functionalist theory of propositional attitudes. The interested reader is referred again to the works cited in note 6.

We are now in a position to sharpen up the foregoing characterization of functionalism. Using the notion of a Ramsey functional correlate, we can express the core doctrine of functionalism as follows: Where ψ is any psychological property, there exists a psychological theory P such that for some i, ψ is identical with the ith Ramsey functional correlate of P.

We are also in a position to distinguish between the two main forms of functionalism.

The first form is a theory that is often called *analytic functionalism.* Analytic functionalists start by giving an account of the semantic properties of our commonsense psychological items, an account that claims that these terms get their meanings from a commonsense theory of mind generally known as *folk psychology.* They then point out that the foregoing doctrine – the core doctrine of functionalism – follows from their semantic hypotheses.

Folk psychology is a set of lawlike generalizations that link psychological terms to one another and to terms of three other kinds – terms that stand for distal stimuli, terms that stand for sensory inputs, and terms that stand for behavioral outputs. Here is a list of sample generalizations collected by Paul Churchland:[8]

Persons tend to feel pain at points of recent bodily damage. (4)

Persons denied fluids tend to feel thirst. (5)

Persons who engage in vigorous activity tend to feel fatigue. (6)

Given normal attention and background conditions, persons tend to perceive many of the observable features of their immediate environment. (7)

Persons in pain tend to want to relieve that pain. (8)

Persons who feel thirst tend to desire potable fluids. (9)

Persons who are angry tend to be impatient. (10)

Persons who are angry tend to frown. (11)

Persons subject to a sudden sharp pain tend to wince and/or cry out. (12)

---

8 Paul Churchland, *Scientific Realism and the Plasticity of Mind* (Cambridge: Cambridge University Press, 1979). I have added a couple of laws to Churchland's list.

Persons who believe that p, where p obviously entails q, tend to believe q.

(13)

Persons who believe that p tend to assent to p when queried. (14)

Barring preferred strategies and/or incompatible desires, persons who desire that p and who believe that q would be sufficient to bring it about that p, tend to desire that q. (15)

If a person desires that q, believes that p would be sufficient for q, and is able to bring it about that p, then, barring preferred strategies and/or incompatible desires, he/she will try to bring it about that p. (16)

Persons who desire that p tend to be pleased if they discover that p is true. (17)

Persons who fear that p tend to want it to be the case that not-p. (18)

Analytic functionalism claims that our commonsense psychological terms get their meanings from laws like these. (If these laws are to serve our present purposes, the term "person" must be understood in a special way. Instead of taking it as a term for members of the biological category homo sapiens, we must see it as a synonym for an expression like "being which is either a member of homo sapiens or roughly similar to members of homo sapiens in behavior and internal architecture." If we were to think of "person" as having a narrower sense in 4–18, we would have to think of 4–18 as constraining the meanings of our psychological terms in such a way as to make it inappropriate to ascribe the terms to androids and members of other biological species. But then we would be unable to see them as providing an adequate basis for analytic functionalism.)

The claim that our commonsense psychological terms get their meanings from the laws of folk psychology leaves some important questions open. It tells us something about the provenience of the meanings of these terms, but it does not tell us much about the meanings themselves. However, analytic functionalists are concerned to analyze these meanings. They do so by appealing to the Ramsey functional descriptions that are associated with folk psychology. Where T is any commonsense psychological term, T will of course be embedded in folk psychology, and it will therefore be the case that there is a Ramsey functional description (associated with folk psychology) that corresponds to T. Analytic functionalists maintain that T is synonymous with the corresponding description. This is the key thesis of analytic functionalism. (Analytic functionalists sometimes prefer to express the thesis by saying that the identity statement that links T to the corresponding Ramsey functional description is a conceptual truth.)

The proposition that I have just called the key thesis of analytic functionalism does not imply the proposition that I earlier called the core doctrine of functionalism – the proposition that where ψ is any psychological property, there exists a psychological theory P such that for some i, ψ is identical with the ith Ramsey functional correlate of P. It implies only that every psychological property that is recognized by commonsense psychology meets this condition. Analytic functionalists acknowledge that there are psychological properties that are not recognized by commonsense psychology – specifically, they acknowledge that scientific psychology has uncovered (and will continue to uncover) psychological properties that are altogether beyond the ken of common sense. An analytic functionalist will typically maintain that these properties are identical with the Ramsey functional correlates of scientific psychological theories.

The second main form of functionalism is generally known as *psychofunctionalism*. Advocates of this view maintain that it is a mistake to identify psychological properties with the Ramsey functional correlates associated with folk psychology, but they assert that such properties can be identified with the Ramsey functional correlates associated with a scientific theory of mind – in particular, with the Ramsey functional correlates of some fully developed version of contemporary cognitive psychology.

There are three main differences between analytic functionalism and psychofunctionalism.

First and foremost, analytic functionalism is a theory of the meanings or *senses* of our commonsense psychological terms; it is a semantic theory, but a semantic theory that has important metaphysical consequences. Psychofunctionalism is not a semantic theory. It asserts that our commonsense psychological expressions refer to or express the same properties as the expressions of some down-the-road psychological theory, but it denies that the former expressions have the same senses as the latter. According to psychofunctionalists, the relationship between a term like "pain" and its counterpart in scientific psychology is like the relationship between "heat" and "average kinetic energy of molecules." The latter expressions can be said to stand for the same property, but they have virtually nothing in common at the level of sense.

Second, analytic functionalists maintain that the core doctrine of functionalism is a conceptual truth, and that it can be seen to be true by a priori analysis. (Strictly speaking, they maintain that this holds for that part of the core doctrine that applies to commonsense psychological properties.) Psychofunctionalists deny this contention. They maintain that functionalism has the status of a high-level scientific hypothesis, and that the task of assessing it is largely empirical.

Third, in analyzing commonsense psychological properties, analytic functionalists are limited to functional properties that can be specified using only commonsense terms for inputs and outputs, but psychofunctionalists are under no such restriction. For example, because we have no commonsense terms for the pathways by which signals enter and depart from the brain stem, the analytic functionalist is precluded from referring to these pathways in analyzing pain. But the psychofunctionalist is not.[9]

III

Although functionalism is currently held in high esteem by the overwhelming majority of professional philosophers, it is open to a number

9 A final point about the content of functionalism. Although the account given in the text is virtually identical to the canonical accounts that are put forward by functionalists, it suffers from a fairly serious flaw. In order to render the account consistent with functionalist views about the distribution of sensations, it is necessary to revise the definition of "Ramsey functional description." To give an adequate definition it is necessary to take account of the fact that the relevant psychological theories will contain universal quantifiers that range over universes of discourse that are highly heterogeneous. (Recall that all occurrences of the implicitly quantificational term "persons" in the laws of folk psychology range over human beings and also over all other creatures who are roughly similar to us in behavioral capacities and internal architecture.)

We can accommodate this fact by stipulating that these universal quantifiers should precede the strings of property-quantifiers I have expressed by "there exist state-types $X_1, \ldots, X_n$ such that." Without some such change, a functional description will carry the presupposition that there exist certain state-types that are common to all members of the universe of discourse of the theory from which the description is derived. That is, it will presuppose that the state-types that occupy a given set of functional roles in the members of one subclass of the universe of discourse are identical with the state-types that occupy those roles in any other subclass. Functionalists cannot allow a functional description to carry this presupposition, for it is incompatible with their doctrine of the multiple realizability of functional roles.

Loar has a different solution. (See Loar, op. cit., pp. 48–49.) In my judgment, both solutions can be made to work.

of objections. In this section and the next I will sketch eight objections – three to analytic functionalism and five to psychofunctionalism. For the most part, the core ideas of the objections will be familiar to those who are acquainted with the literature – though the slant is different in some cases, and in other cases there is supplementary argumentation that goes beyond what has been said elsewhere.

Does the popularity of functionalism show that the familiar objections are weak or irrelevant? Not in my view; in my view the familiar objections are extremely strong. If they have thus far failed to cause a general turning away from functionalism, this is due in part to the fact that they have not always been formulated in a fully adequate way. Moreover, it appears to be true that we are normally willing to overlook the flaws of a theory, even if they are extremely serious, until we have been presented with a viable alternative. We tend to cling to old beliefs until we find new beliefs that can serve as replacements. Assuming that this is true, and assuming also that the present work offers a reasonably good case for the proposition that type materialism is a viable alternative to functionalism, it may be that the familiar objections will have a greater appeal in the present context than they have had in others.

I will now state the objections to *analytic* functionalism that seem to me to have the greatest force.

1. One of the primary forces moving the inventors of analytic functionalism was the intuition that our psychological concepts can be applied to beings who differ radically from ourselves and also from one another both in internal structure and in material composition. The first objection, often called the *absent qualia argument*, charges that the inventors overestimated the scope of this intuition. It charges that they were misled by the intuition into representing the scope of our concepts as being substantially broader than it actually is.

The most vivid and powerful version of the objection is due to Ned Block.[10] Block invites us to imagine a being who is quite different than we are at a cellular level. Instead of being composed of neurons, the "brain" of the creature consists of homunculi who communicate with one another by radio. However, there is a one-to-one correspondence between these homunculi and the neurons of a typical human being, and

---

10 See Block, "Troubles with Functionalism" in his anthology, *Readings in the Philosophy of Psychology*, Vol. I (Cambridge, Mass.: Harvard University Press, 1980), 268–305. The most relevant passages occur in sections 1.2–1.5.

the transmission of inhibitory and excitatory signals is preserved perfectly by the correspondence. As a result, the being is isomorphic to ourselves at all supracellular levels of internal organization. Moreover, it has exactly the same behavioral capacities.

Now analytic functionalism implies that this creature has exactly the same psychological states as we do. It has beliefs and desires, it has emotions and moods, and it has sensations. But this consequence seems highly questionable, to say the least! After all, the homunculi Block imagines are just like ourselves except in size. The idea that the activities of a group of such beings could give birth to consciousness seems perfectly wild!

In thinking through the details of this example, it is important to distinguish between the conscious experiences that belong to the Blockean homunculi and the conscious experiences that are attributed by functionalism to the being who is composed of the homunculi. There is a sense in which it is trivially true that a group of Blockean homunculi can give birth to consciousness: The group as a whole can be said to give birth to the set (or the logical fusion) of the conscious experiences that are associated respectively with the individual members of the group. But this set (or fusion) is entirely distinct from the conscious experiences that functionalism attributes to the larger being. To underscore this fact, we could imagine that the conscious experiences of the larger being are qualitatively different from those of the beings who serve as his constituents. (He feels pain even when they feel pleasure, and so on.)

Perhaps it will be useful to give the absent qualia argument a second formulation. According to analytic functionalism, it is conceptually true that pain is identical with the functional state that is picked out by a certain folk-psychological description (hereafter called "description D"). Hence, analytic functionalism implies that whenever we conceive of a creature as being in a state that is picked out by description D, we are fully committed to conceiving of the creature as being in pain. But this consequence is false. We can see that it is false by conceiving of a homunculi-headed robot whose brain is isomorphic to a typical human brain. A robot of this sort is fully capable of being in the state that is picked out by description D. Accordingly, if analytic functionalism were true, we would be committed to the view that such beings have the capacity to feel pain. That is to say, if analytic functionalism were true, then, after reflecting on the similarities between such beings and ourselves, and adjusting to the differences, we would embrace this view. However, it seems that our primary response to the view, both before and after reflection, is negative. We are much more strongly inclined to reject the view than to embrace it.

Generalizing this point, we can say that analytic functionalism must be rejected because it fails to predict or explain our dispositions to ascribe terms like "pain" and "itch" to other beings. According to analytic functionalism, our willingness to ascribe such terms to another being depends entirely or almost entirely on the functional organization of the being. But this is false. We can know that the functional organization of a being is the same as ours and still be unwilling to use the terms in describing the being's internal states.

There are four complaints about the absent qualia argument that must now be considered.

First complaint. As Block himself has pointed out, it can seem absurd to suppose that collections of neurons are capable of sustaining qualitative states. That is to say, we have intuitions about brain states that parallel our intuitions about the activities of homunculi: "Is a hunk of quivering gray stuff more intuitively appropriate as a seat of qualia than a covey of little men?"[11] Because we know that our intuitions about brain states are wrong, perhaps we should discount all intuitions that belong to the same category – including our negative intuitions about Blockean homunculi-heads. Perhaps there is something inherently untrustworthy about the members of this category.

Reply. The question of whether we feel comfortable about ascribing qualitative states to brain-headed creatures is a red herring. Analytic functionalism predicts that we will ascribe such states to all creatures who have a certain functional organization. As we can see from reflecting on Blockean homunculi-heads, this prediction is false. Period. The fact that we sometimes feel uncomfortable about ascribing qualitative states to non-Blockean beings who have that organization (namely, ourselves) tends to strengthen the case against analytic functionalism, not to weaken it.

Second complaint. It is perhaps true that we can conceive of a creature that has the functional organization of a human being while lacking qualitative states, but how could this fact impugn the thesis that mental states are identical with functional properties? We can conceive of many things that we know to be absurd – for example, a collection of H_2O molecules that does not count as a case of water. What we can conceive of is one thing; what is true is another.

11 See Block, ibid., p. 281.

Reply. It must be acknowledged that there is a strong prima facie case against arguing from premises about conceivability to conclusions about reality. However, we can acknowledge this while endorsing the absent qualia argument. It is crucial to remember here that analytic functionalists are not content to make a factual claim. According to them, it is *conceptually* true that psychological properties are identical with functional properties. In saying this, they give us license to appeal to data about conceivability in testing their views. Even if it is a mistake to use such data in testing factual claims, it is entirely legitimate to do so when one is assessing a conceptual claim.

To be sure, it is necessary to proceed with caution even when we are using facts about conceivability in connection with assessments of this second kind. We must take steps to ensure that our conceptualizations are clear and distinct, and we must also make sure that our conceptualizations satisfy certain standards of completeness. But it is clear that we can construct Blockean counterexamples to analytic functionalism that fulfill any reasonable requirements of this sort. We can build a virtually limitless amount of information into our conceptualization of Blockean homunculi-heads without reducing their effectiveness as counterexamples. We can build in information about their structure, composition, and origin – information of any sort that might be thought relevant to the enterprise of making third-person ascriptions of pain. And, having done so, we will still be unwilling to say that homunculi-heads are capable of being in pain.

Third complaint. If it is false, as the objection maintains, that homunculi-heads can experience pain, then it must also be false that homunculi-heads can be in a state that is functionally equivalent to pain. For a state to be functionally equivalent to pain, the state must have a tendency to cause the same beliefs and desires that pain has a tendency to cause. However, beliefs and desires are individuated by the contents of their constituent concepts. Hence, to have the same beliefs and desires as we do, a homunculi-head would have to have a concept with the same content as our concept of pain. But this is impossible if it is true that homunculi-heads are incapable of experiencing pain. For our concept of pain gets its content from certain causal relations between pain itself and internal states of which the concept is a constituent. (Thus, the content of the concept derives in part from the fact that states of pain can cause us to form the belief that we are currently experiencing pain.)

Reply. This complaint can be deflected by rephrasing the first objection as a dilemma: Either homunculi-heads are capable of forming a concept with the same content as our concept of pain or they are not. If they are, then the objection goes through in its original form. If they are not, then it must be the case that the content of our concept of pain derives from causal relations between states involving the concept (beliefs, and so on) and certain features of states of pain, where the features in question are not present in the corresponding states of homunculi-heads. Specifically, it must be the case that the content of the concept of pain derives from causal relations between states involving the concept of pain and *intrinsic* features of states of pain. So we reach the conclusion that the content of our concept of pain must derive from the intrinsic nature of pain. But then analytic functionalism is wrong; for it claims that the content of our concept of pain derives from its role in a commonsense psychological theory.[12]

Fourth complaint. The behavior of a homunculi-head depends on the intentions of its constituent homunculi, and these intentions could change at any moment. After all, even if they are very small, people have free will! The homunculi would decide to go on strike! Hence, a homunculi-head does not satisfy the same behavioral counterfactuals as a human being. And this implies that the internal states of a homunculi-head do not have the same functional roles as our internal states.

Reply. Imagine that the homunculi have been hypnotized, or that they have taken a mind-constraining drug.

2. According to our first objection to analytic functionalism, it is possible to conceive of instances of functional properties that fail to exemplify the corresponding qualitative characteristics. The second objection puts forward the converse of this claim. It affirms that we can conceive of instances of qualitative characteristics that fail to exemplify the corresponding functional properties.

Because the main point of this objection is the converse of the main point of the absent qualia argument, it is natural to refer to the objection as the *absent functional role argument* (or the *absent role argument*, for short).

---

12 Why must we say that the content of the concept of pain derives from causal relations between states involving the concept and intrinsic features of states of pain? Why not say instead that the content of the concept of pain derives from causal relations between states involving the concept of pain and functional properties of states of pain?

    If the content of the concept of pain derives from the functional properties of states of pain, then the content of the concept of pain would derive from features that are also present in the corresponding states of homunculi-heads, and so, contrary to hypothesis, Blockean homunculi-heads would have the same concept of pain as we do.

I am now attending to an itch in my left leg. This itch has several properties of the sort that functionalists are wont to emphasize. In particular, it has the power to make me want to scratch my left leg. This property is easily the most distinctive of the functional properties that the itch exemplifies. Hence, if any functional property is definitive of the property *being an itch*, this one is. However, I can easily conceive of a sensation that has the same intrinsic nature as my present itch and that lacks this functional property. Moreover, when I conceive of a sensation of this sort, I find that it seems entirely appropriate to ascribe the term "itch" to it. As long as I conceive of a sensation as having the same intrinsic nature as the sensation in my left leg, the former sensation has as strong a claim on the term "itch" as the latter.

When I urge that it is possible to conceive of events that exemplify qualitative characteristics without exemplifying the functional properties that normally accompany those characteristics, I sometimes meet with great resistance. But actually, we have reason to believe that there are events that meet this condition even in the actual world. We are all aware that victims of paralysis can experience many of the same sensations as the rest of us. The sensations of these individuals tend to have causal and counterfactual relations to other *internal* phenomena that are perfectly standard, but it is nonetheless true that their functional properties are quite different from the functional properties that other sensations exemplify. Further, there are individuals who show behavioral signs of having sensations but who lack the conceptual and cognitive capacities that the rest of us enjoy. Consider a person whose capacities have been severely eroded by Alzheimer's disease. Or consider a fetus. Or even a young baby. It is clear that a baby can have sensations, but can a baby have beliefs about sensations? Can a baby remember sensations? Can a baby desire that a sensation cease? Few of us would be inclined to give affirmative answers to these questions. But then we are committed to denying that the sensations of babies are causally and counterfactually related to other internal phenomena in the standard ways.

In view of these considerations, it seems that we should be disposed to embrace the absent role argument with enthusiasm. Yet, as I said, the argument is often resisted. I think that the resistance has two sources.

First, I think that people have a tendency to build too much into the imaginative pictures they construct in the course of considering the argument. They form imaginative pictures of situations in which they themselves – or beings like themselves – are attending to itches or pains. It is not surprising that these pictures tend to give rise to functionalist intuitions. If one imagines a situation in which there is an itch and *an owner* of that itch who is pretty much like oneself, then one will inevitably think that the itch has a tendency to produce the desire to scratch. But this is only because the itch is represented as occurring in a being who is disposed to want to scratch itches! If one imagines the itch as occurring in a being of a different kind, one will reach a quite different conclusion.

Second, I think that functionalists may sometimes reason as follows. In order to appreciate the merits of analytic functionalism, we must distinguish between the claim that itches cause one to desire to scratch and the claim that itches have a tendency to cause one to have this desire. Analytic functionalism asserts that the latter claim is a conceptual truth, but it does not maintain that the former claim has this status. Accordingly, analytic functionalism cannot be refuted by pointing out that it is possible to conceive of a sensation that exemplifies *being an itch* but that is not accompanied by a desire to scratch. To show that analytic functionalism is false, it is necessary to conceive of a sensation that exemplifies *being an itch* but that is not of a kind such that members of that kind have a tendency to cause one to desire to scratch. But it is impossible to conceive of an itch of this sort. To be sure, it can seem that we are doing so. However, if we attend carefully to the state we are in when we are under the impression that we are conceiving of such an itch, we will find that the impression is mistaken. We will find that we believe, at least implicitly, that the itch we are considering is the kind of thing that has a tendency to cause us to desire to scratch. Because of this belief, it is true to say that we are conceiving of the itch in terms of the tendency to cause a desire to scratch. And by the same token, it is true to say that we are conceiving of it as having a functional property.

It might be said, in response to this line of thought, that the belief in question is not internally related to the state of conceiving of an itch – that the belief merely accompanies one's representation of the itch, without in any sense being a constituent of it, and that it therefore has no bearing on the question of how we conceive of the itch. I will, however, waive this objection and confine myself to pointing out that, contrary to what the line of thought maintains, the property attributed by the belief is not a functional property. Let us conceive of a sensation that has the intrinsic nature that is peculiar to itches; but let us conceive of it as belonging to someone who does not have the normal neural architecture, and who, as a result, is incapable of desiring to scratch. Let us call this sensation "Ishmael." Now it may well be the case that we believe, at least implicitly, that Ishmael is the kind of thing that has a tendency to cause a desire to scratch. But do we mean to be attributing a functional property to Ishmael by this belief? It seems that the answer must be "no." As can be seen from the foregoing exposition of functionalism, if a sensation has a given functional property, it must exemplify a state-type λ such that λ occupies the functional role that corresponds to that functional property *in the being in whom that sensation occurs* (and in other beings of the same kind). Hence, if we meant to be attributing a functional property to Ishmael, we would have to think that Ishmael exemplifies a state-type that plays a certain functional role in the being in whom Ishmael occurs – the role that itches play in beings that are capable of desiring to scratch. However, we would have to be extremely confused to think that; for by hypothesis, Ishmael does not exemplify a state-type that plays this role in the being in which Ishmael occurs. Because it seems that we are able to conceive of Ishmael, and to hold the belief in question (the belief that Ishmael is the kind of thing that has a tendency to cause a desire to scratch), without being extremely confused, it seems quite unlikely that we mean, in holding the belief, to be attributing a functional property to Ishmael.

All things considered, it seems reasonable to suppose that the belief in question is concerned with the following property: *being an instance of a state-type ϕ such that instances of ϕ that occur in normal beings have a tendency to cause a desire to scratch*. This is not a property of the sort that analytic functionalists claim to be constitutive of *being an itch*. It is not a functional property. Ishmael exemplifies the property by virtue of standing in a relation (the relation *being an instance of the same state-type as*) to sensations that occur in beings with normal neural architecture, and that are able to cause a desire to scratch because they occur in such beings. In other words, Ishmael has the property because Ishmael exemplifies a state-type that occupies a certain functional role in beings that are quite different than the being in which Ishmael occurs. (The state-type in question does not occupy this role in the latter being.) But a functional property is not a property that something can have simply by virtue of exemplifying a state-type that occupies a functional role in beings of some kind or other. As we just noticed, if a property counts as functional, it is impossible for a state-token to exemplify that property unless the token exemplifies a state-type that occupies an appropriate functional role in beings of the same kind as the "owner" of the token.

It is easy to see why someone might be tempted by the line of thought of two paragraphs ago. Suppose that a certain functional property is defined by saying that its instances have a tendency to cause phenomena of type ψ. Suppose also that a certain state-type, ϕ, occupies the functional role that corresponds to this property in beings of type β. Here it can be extremely tempting to think that all instances of ϕ are instances of the functional property – even those instances that occur in beings of a different kind. After all, one is inclined to think, the functional property is defined in terms of a tendency. It follows that the connection between the property and ψ is loose and probabilistic, and it follows from this in turn that instances of ϕ that occur in beings of type β can exemplify the functional property even if they are not accompanied by instances of ψ. Perhaps it even follows that there can be beings of type β such that (1) instances of ϕ that occur in those beings exemplify the functional property even though (2) such instances are never accompanied by instances of ψ. So why not say that instances of ϕ can exemplify the functional property even when they occur in beings in which instances of ψ *cannot* occur?

Although it is natural to ask this question, it betrays a confusion about the notion of a functional property. It presupposes that a state-token that occurs in a being of one kind can be said to exemplify a functional property merely by virtue of exemplifying a state-type that plays a certain functional role in beings of a different kind. As we just noticed, however, this presupposition is wrong. Functional properties are limited to properties that tokens exemplify by virtue of exemplifying state-types that occupy functional roles in the beings in which the tokens occur.

3. My third objection to analytic functionalism stems from an epistemological point. (Accordingly, it might be called the *epistemological argument*.) The point can be expressed by saying that it is the immediately perceived intrinsic nature of a state-token that justifies one in ascribing a term like "itch" or "pain" to the token.

What justifies me in ascribing "pain" to one of my own sensations? There may be indirect evidence of one sort or another. For example, I may have just determined, by using an autocerebroscope, that I am presently in the brain state that has always accompanied pain in the past. However, the best and most fundamental justification for ascribing "pain" to a state-token is the fact that the token exemplifies *being a pain*. In other words, it seems that we should accept (19):

> In order to be strongly justified in believing that one is in pain, it is enough that one be in a sensory state that exemplifies *being a pain*. (19)

(19) is supported by certain of our intuitions about justification. (I will say more in defense of (19) in section V of Chapter 5.)

65

Now it seems that (19) is incompatible with analytic functionalism. Thus, according to analytic functionalism, it is conceptually true that pain is identical with the property *being a state-token y such that y is a P*, where "*being a state-token y such that y is a P*" abbreviates a Ramsey functional description that is based on folk psychology. Further, it is evident that the following principle is correct: If one has grounds that strongly justify one in believing that *p*, and it is conceptually true that if *p* then *q*, then it is possible to come to see, by reflecting on the content of the relevant concepts, that one's grounds for believing that *p* are also grounds that strongly justify one in believing that *q*. It follows that if one has grounds that strongly justify one in believing that one has a pain, then it is possible to come to see, by reflecting on the contents of the relevant concepts, that these grounds strongly justify one in believing that one has a sensation that exemplifies *being a state-token y such that y is a P*. When this proposition is combined with (19), we get the result that it is possible to see that the nature of one of one's sensations can strongly justify one in believing that one has a sensation that exemplifies *being a state-token y such that y is a P*. But this result is absurd. In effect, all of folk psychology is built into the description that is abbreviated by "*being a state-token y such that y is a P*." Hence, if one believes that one of one's sensations exemplifies *being a state-token y such that y is a P*, then one has a belief that in effect presupposes the truth of folk psychology. That is to say, one has a belief that in effect presupposes the truth of an extremely complicated empirical theory – a theory that makes a large number of rather strong claims about the functional architecture of human beings and about the etiology of human behavior. It could not possibly be the case that one was strongly justified in holding a belief of this sort solely on the basis of information about the nature of a single sensation. Rather, one's justification must include information to the effect that folk psychology has enjoyed a considerable amount of success in the past – success in predicting and explaining a wide variety of mental states, and in predicting and explaining a wide variety of actions.

To be sure, we do sometimes say that a single experience justifies us in ascribing a complex theoretical property to something. Thus, we might say that the experience of seeing a light in the sky justifies us in ascribing the property *being an interior planet of the sun* to the entity that is the source of the light. But in saying this we do not mean to say that the ascription is strongly justified by the experience. (If we describe the experience as *the* justification for ascribing the property, we mean only that it is the most salient part of the justification.) A strong justification would have to include the body of evidence – perhaps evidence deriving from the testimony of others, perhaps evidence that we have obtained ourselves – that gives us the right to embrace the propositions of astronomy that are presupposed by our ascription.

IV

Before I turn to the task of assessing psychofunctionalism, I will make a few additional observations about the content of this theory, and a few remarks about the constraints that objections must satisfy in order to count as relevant.

A state of affairs is said to be *logically possible* if it is compatible with all of the logical truths, with all of the conceptual truths, and with all of the truths that belong to certain related categories (such as the category of mathematical truths). On the other hand, a state of affairs is said to be *nomologically* (or *physically*) *possible* if it is logically possible and it is compatible with all of the laws of nature. It follows, of course, that the nomologically possible states of affairs are a proper subset of the logically possible state of affairs.

This classification of states of affairs induces a classification of possible worlds. A possible world counts as logically possible if all of its constituent states of affairs are logically possible, and as nomologically possible if all of its constituent states of affairs are nomologically possible. It follows that the class of nomologically possible worlds is properly included in the class of logically possible worlds. (For these explanations to work, we need to adopt the view that the states of affairs that are constituents of a given possible world include all of the states of affairs that are (finite or infinite) conjunctions of other constituents of that world. Otherwise there would be a problem about *compossibility*.)

Now, where ψ is a qualitative characteristic, psychofunctionalists wish to identify ψ with the property of being a state-token x such that x exemplifies a state-type that plays the role associated with ψ in the members of some category of beings. We must now ask: Which state-tokens are relevant here? Does the relevant class consist of all of the tokens that satisfy the given condition in any logically possible worlds? Or does it consist only of tokens that satisfy the condition in nomologically possible worlds? Or does it consist of tokens that are found in the members of some third category of worlds?

It seems that we can rule out the first option immediately. Suppose that ϕ is the property that psychofunctionalists wish to identify with pain. If

67

every state-token whatsoever could count as an instance of ϕ, no matter how bizarre, provided only that it exemplifies a type that plays the appropriate functional role in some logically possible world, then ϕ would have instances that involve the activities of groups of Blockean homunculi. For even though Blockean homunculi-heads cannot be found in nomologically possible worlds, they are rife in worlds that lie beyond the realm of nomological possibility. The moral is obvious: If psychofunctionalists were to avail themselves of the first option, then their position would collapse into analytic functionalism, and it would be possible to refute them by the foregoing absent qualia argument.

On the other hand, it seems reasonable to suppose that psychofunctionalists want the instances of ϕ to include every token of a type that plays the appropriate role in some nomologically possible world. For it is one of their primary contentions that various beings who *could* be created by scientists are sentient. This group includes a wide range of biological beings (beings who could be produced by genetic engineering), and also a large variety of beings who do not fall under the laws of biology (such as silicon-based androids). (A terminological aside: In the sequel I will use "nonbiological android" as an abbreviation for "android whose physical composition is quite different from that of human beings." (This might suggest that Blockean homunculi-heads should count as biological androids; for *ex hypothesi* they are composed of flesh and blood. However, because their existence is not compatible with the laws of biology, I do not wish to classify Blockean homunculi-heads as biological beings. A biological android is a flesh-and-blood android whose existence is compatible with the laws of biology.)

Perhaps there are psychofunctionalists who would like ϕ to have instances in some worlds that are not nomologically possible. There are various belts of worlds that extend beyond the belt of nomological possibility but do not extend all the way to the outer fringes of logical possibility. Perhaps there are psychofunctionalists who would like to define ϕ over the worlds in one of these other belts. However, I know of no public pronouncements to this effect. Accordingly, it is not unreasonable to interpret psychofunctionalists as holding that the instances of ϕ include all and only those tokens that exemplify types that play the appropriate role in nomologically possible worlds. I will call this the *minimal* interpretation.

The admissibility of the minimal interpretation has an important methodological implication. Because it is admissible, if one wishes to give a counterexample that calls psychofunctionalism into question on all admissible interpretations, one must select an example from the actual world or some other world in the belt of nomological possibility. Information about worlds outside this belt is not relevant. Thus, for example, if one wishes to give a counterexample in which the functional correlate of *being a pain* is exemplified but in which *being a pain* is not, one must try to find a case that meets this condition in the actual world or in some other nomologically possible world.[13]

Having taken note of these points, we are in a position to consider some objections to psychofunctionalism. I will present five.

1. My first objection calls attention to an important lacuna in psychofunctionalism. I call it the *semantic complaint.*

Psychofunctionalists have thus far been content to put forward a metaphysical claim about the nature of psychological properties – specifically, the claim that each psychological property is identical with a Ramsey functional correlate of some yet-to-be-discovered psychological theory. It is apparent, however, that this is not enough. Psychofunctionalists also have an obligation to show that this metaphysical claim is compatible with a well-motivated account of the meanings of psychological terms. For example, they must explain how it is possible for me to use "pain" to refer to a property that lies far beyond my ken – a property that is one of the Ramsey functional correlates of a theory that I do not know and that in all likelihood cannot even be stated without using terms that are foreign to my current vocabulary. The claim that I use "pain" to refer to a property of this sort may not be incoherent or absurd, but it does require explanation and defense.

More: The point is not just that psychofunctionalists owe us a semantic account of "pain" and its affiliates. They owe us an account of a certain kind – namely, an account that is at least as well-motivated and at least as simple as the nonfunctionalist account that I will formulate in Chapter 7.

---

13 This restriction excludes counterexamples involving Blockean homunculi-heads and also counterexamples like the one involving the people of China that Block presents on pp. 276–78 of the paper cited in footnote 10. (Examples of the latter sort are excluded because each of the individuals involved would have to act more rapidly than is nomologically possible in order for the group as a whole to simulate the computational processes of the brain.) The restriction may also exclude counterexamples based on spectrum inversion. We simply do not know enough at present to be able to say whether the relevant sort of spectrum inversion is nomologically possible. (The relevant sort is the sort that Lycan calls "inversion with respect to input–output relations *plus* internal functional organization." See William G. Lycan, *Consciousness* (Cambridge, MA: MIT Press, 1987), p. 60.)

Although I think there are grounds for doubt as to whether it is possible for psychofunctionalists to satisfy this criterion, I will not attempt to detail these grounds here. (It will, I think, become apparent what they are when the reader gets to Chapter 7.) Instead, I will just point out that at present there is a hole in psychofunctionalism that one could drive a truck through, and that until they succeed in plugging this hole, it is incumbent on psychofunctionalists to be restrained and tentative in singing the praises of their theory.

2. The second objection is closely related to the first of the foregoing objections to analytic functionalism. Accordingly, despite certain differences that will soon become apparent, I will call this objection the *second absent qualia argument*.

The objection derives from two claims. First, there is the claim that insofar as we are free from superstition and conceptual confusion, our willingness to attribute sensations to other beings, whether the beings are actual or possible, varies directly with our perceptions concerning the similarities between the other beings and ourselves. Second, there is the claim that the relevant similarities include similarities that are nonfunctional – that is, the claim that we must believe the other beings to resemble us in point of any nonfunctional properties that can reasonably be thought to have something to do with the occurrence of sensory states in human beings. These claims are controversial, but it is nonetheless true that they can be seen to be correct by reflecting on our intuitions about concrete cases. Thus, the first claim is strongly supported by the fact that we *would* be willing to ascribe sensations to Blockean homunculi-heads if we believed that *our own brains* were composed of homunculi. If we were given evidence that led us to believe that we were homunculi-heads ourselves, and that led us to believe that our sensations were in some way dependent on the activities of our constituent homunculi (in the way that we now believe that our sensations are in some way dependent on the activities of our constituent neurons), we would be willing to see Blockean androids as sentient beings. It is reasonable to conclude from this that our reluctance – in the actual situation, the situation that is defined in part by our belief that our sensations depend in some way on the activities of neurons – to attribute sensations to Blockean androids is due to the fact that such androids are quite different from ourselves. As for the second claim, to see its merits, we need only recall that Blockean androids are identical to us in functional properties. This indicates that our reluctance to ascribe sensations to them is due to the fact that we believe them to be quite different from ourselves at nonfunctional levels of description.

Assuming that the two claims are correct, we can see that psycho-functionalists must be wrong in asserting that we are committed to attributing sensations to nonbiological androids. After all, nonbiological androids are no less different from us than Blockean homunculi-heads. Moreover, they differ from us in much the same way as Blockean homunculi-heads.

To heighten our appreciation of these differences, let us consider a silicon-based android who is maximally similar to human beings. Specifically, let us consider one whose brain is as close as possible to being isomorphic – at all supracellular levels – to the human brain. This brain must of course consist of artificial neurons, but we can imagine that it is housed in a normal human body, and that things have been set up in such a way that the artificial neurons can receive signals from the afferent neurons in the body and can also send (highly efficacious) commands to the efferent neurons. Let us call this being "C4PO."

Even though C4PO is maximally similar to a normal human being, the differences are enormous. First, C4PO's neurons differ radically from ours both in internal structure and in material composition. Second, the laws that govern the behavior of C4PO's artificial neurons are quite different from the laws that govern the behavior of real neurons: Among other things, C4PO's neurons require different forms and sources of energy, and they operate much more rapidly. (Unless C4PO's designer has taken steps to counteract the rapidity with which the neurons operate, there will inevitably be significant differences between C4PO's behavior and the behavior of the average person. On the other hand, if the designer has compensated for this rapidity by building delay elements into the individual neurons, the internal structural differences must be even greater than we have already imagined them to be.)

Because of these considerations, I find that I am unwilling to attribute sensations to C4PO. But functionalists do not share this attitude. Instead of refusing to ascribe sensations to creatures like C4PO, they maintain that it is obvious that such creatures can have sensations, and they claim that it is one of the cardinal virtues of their theory that it preserves and explains this perception. What is going on here? Are we confronted with a difference in intuitions that is so deep as to be beyond resolution? Perhaps. But there is an alternative explanation that I prefer. There are various considerations that count in favor of attributing sensations to creatures like C4PO, and various considerations that counsel against this move. I think that functionalists have overestimated the importance of a consideration that belongs to the first group.

The consideration I have in mind can be expressed as follows: If we were in a situation in which we interacted with highly developed androids on a daily basis, we would inevitably come to use the language of folk psychology in explaining their behavior. That is to say, we would use terms like "belief," "desire," and "intention" in explaining their behavior, and terms like "taste of onions," "itch," and "pain" as well. We would have no choice. The vocabulary of folk psychology is the only part of our everyday conceptual scheme that would provide an adequate basis for explanations.

It seems likely to me that functionalists are inclined to view this fact about our linguistic dispositions as having supreme importance, but I think that this view is wrong. Although the fact is obviously an important consideration, it does not show that we are committed to regarding androids as sentient beings. To see the merits of this claim, observe that we would find ourselves inexorably drawn to using the language of folk psychology if we were in a situation in which we interacted on a daily basis with Blockean homunculi-heads. We would be forced to use terms like "belief" and "pain" in giving explanations of their behavior. However, with the exception of a few diehard fans of analytic functionalism, it is acknowledged on all sides that it is highly counterintuitive to say that Blockean beings can have pains in the literal sense of "pain." Indeed, it is in part because this is so counterintuitive that psychofunctionalists prefer their position to that of the analytic functionalists.

As I see it, then, there are cases that show that we can be disposed to ascribe the term "pain" to the members of a group of creatures without being disposed to regard those creatures as genuinely sentient beings. That is to say, there are situations in which we would freely use "pain" in giving explanations of behavior, but in which we would be using the term (no doubt without fully realizing it) in an extended sense. Before we can appropriately conclude that a creature is in pain in the literal sense of the term, we must have reason to believe that the creature is similar to ourselves at a very deep level. And nonbiological androids – even very complicated ones – fail to satisfy this requirement.

When psychofunctionalists consider silicon-based androids, they allow their intuitions about sentience to be dictated by linguistic dispositions. But they are able to resist this temptation when they consider Blockean homunculi-heads. Why? What is the explanation of this difference? I think they are inclined to view silicon-based androids as sentient because they are aware that daily interaction with relatively simple androids of this sort could become a reality in the not-too-distant future, and they already feel the anticipatory stirrings of their own linguistic dispositions. Like the rest of us, they frequently encounter such androids in the pages of science fiction novels and in the prophesies of futurologists. When they do so, they *experience* the inevitability of using terms like "pain" in accounting for the behavior of such creatures. They view the androids through a screen of partially activated linguistic dispositions. On the other hand, because there is no chance whatsoever that Blockean beings will someday come into existence, the apprehension that we would have to use terms like "pain" in accounting for behavior of such beings is purely intellectual. It is possible to be objective in this case because the question of sentience is not prejudged by anticipatory responses.

Two final points.

First, terms tend to acquire new senses when they are used metaphorically over a period of time. A use that starts life as a metaphor may wind up as literally correct. It seems likely that this fate would befall the language of folk psychology if we were to interact with androids over a period of time. It would eventually become possible for us to use folk psychological terms in explaining the android's behavior without stretching the meanings of those terms – they would acquire meanings that were appropriate to their new roles. This would of course make it more difficult to realize that there is a philosophical question about the sentience of androids, and it would make it virtually impossible to discuss this question. Fortunately, we may be able to resolve the question before it is swept away by a linguistic tidal wave.

Second, although this is not the place to discuss the issue, we should observe that questions about the moral status of androids are not necessarily settled by our answer to the question of sentience. It is no doubt true that sentience is a necessary condition of certain rights, and perhaps also of certain responsibilities, but it is far from clear that it is a necessary condition of all rights and responsibilities. We might find on reflection that the functional counterparts of sentience are as relevant to some questions about rights and responsibilities as is sentience itself.

3. The third objection is a line of thought that I call the *first heterogeneity argument.*

This objection is based on certain facts about the distribution of sensations within the species homo sapiens. We took note of some of these facts in reflecting on the absent role argument in the previous section. First, as we noticed then, despite the fact that victims of paralysis are incapable of displaying the normal behavioral manifestations of sensations, it is nonetheless appropriate to suppose that they can experience a wide range of sensory states. (Observe in this connection that the impairment of these individuals is not a purely behavioral matter. Typically they are incapable of issuing commands to their muscles. That is to say, not only are there no behavioral outputs, there are no outputs on the exit channels leading from the brain.) Second, as we also noticed, there are individuals – victims of Alzheimer's disease, fetuses, babies, and so on – who present us with plenty of behavioral evidence that they experience sensations, but who are incapable of being in the cognitive and conative states that sensations normally occasion. Third, as is generally known, individuals who have been given certain analgesics (for example, morphine derivatives) report that they continue to experience pain, and even that their pains continue at the same level of intensity, but that their pains no longer bother them. Although there are various ways of explaining their testimony, the most natural way is surely to say that pain is no longer capable of causing the normal affective responses in these individuals, and accordingly that it has lost the major internal component of its normal causal role. Fourth, patients who have undergone lobotomies are sometimes inclined to say things that are similar to these analgesic-occasioned comments. Again, the most natural way of explaining the data is to say that there has been a change in causal role. Finally, pain seems to have different causal roles in certain individuals who are physically similar to the rest of us but whose personalities are somewhat deviant – consider masochists and daredevils.

As I see it, these facts about distribution make it quite likely that qualitative characteristics are not fully coextensive in the members of homo sapiens with the functional properties that accompany them in normal cases. If anything is clear, it is clear that the pains of paralytics and babies differ radically in functional properties from the pains of the rest of us. To be sure, someone might try to accommodate the foregoing cases by maintaining that there is some very abstractly individuated functional property that is common to all cases of pain in the members of homo sapiens. It might be held, for example, that some form of aversion is present in all cases – or that aversion-or-something-like-aversion is always present. However, it seems to me that even this very weak claim is called into qusetion by the foregoing examples. Moreover, even if the claim could be justified, it would fall far short of what the functionalist needs to show – namely, that there is a functional property that accompanies pain in all cases and that is *exemplified only when pain is exemplified*. The more abstractly individuated the functional properties we consider, the less likely it is that they will be present only when pain is present. Thus, for example, aversion is no less likely to accompany nausea or intense itching than to accompany pain.

The present line of thought is closely related to the absent role argument against analytic functionalism. The main point of the absent role argument can be expressed by saying that it is possible to conceive of instances of qualitative characteristics that lack the functional properties with which these characteristics are normally associated. The main point of the first heterogeneity argument is similar. Like the absent role argument, it calls attention to instances of qualitative characteristics that lack the stereotypical functional correlates of the characteristics. It is different only in that the instances to which it refers can all be found in the actual world.

Here someone may object as follows: "You have considered only functional differences that can be picked out by terms that belong to the vocabulary of folk psychology. The existence of functional differences at this level is no guarantee that there are functional differences at deeper levels. In particular, even granting that the claims you have made are correct, it may be true that there are functional similarities at the level that is appropriate to some yet-to-be-discovered psychological theory. And, if this is true, then your claims pose no threat to psychofunctionalism. For psychofunctionalists have long recognized that it may be necessary to identify pain with a functional property that lies far beyond the ken of common sense – that is, with a property that can only be adequately defined from the perspective afforded by a psychological theory that as yet has not even been glimpsed."

Here the objector has missed a key point about the nature of functional roles. It is true that, when seen from the perspective of psychofunctionalism, the functional role of an internal state depends in part on the relations that the state bears to phenomena that lie outside the ken of common sense. However, it is also true that the functional role of a state is largely a matter of relations to phenomena that are fully accessible to common sense – that is, to behavioral phenomena and to introspectible mental phenomena. (How could it be otherwise, given that psychofunctionalism claims that functional roles are to be defined with reference to the laws of a psychological theory, and given also that it is the mission of psychology to provide explanations of behavioral phenomena and of introspectible mental phenomena?) It follows, of course, that if an internal state bears different relations to behaviorial and introspectible phenomena in different subjects, then it occupies different functional roles in those subjects. But we have found that pain can bear quite different relations to behaviorial and introspectible phenomena in different members of *homo sapiens*. Indeed, what is most to the point, we have found that it can occur even in subjects who are *incapable* of displaying normal pain behavior, and even in subjects who are *incapable* of being in some of the introspectible mental states that normally accompany pain. Accordingly, we may conclude that there is no one functional role – nor even a disjunction of similar functional roles – that is invariably correlated with pain in members of *homo sapiens*.

4. As the reader has no doubt anticipated, my fourth objection is called the *second heterogeneity argument*. Whereas the first heterogeneity argument is concerned with the distribution of sensations within the population of human beings, including those who are very young and those who are temporarily or permanently abnormal in some respect or other, the second heterogeneity argument is concerned with the distribution of sensations within the set consisting of normal or representative members of the various animal species.

According to psychofunctionalism, psychological states are individuated in part by the causal and probabilistic relations they bear to other psychological states. It follows from this that psychological states come in systems, or constellations: To be capable of being in a given psychological state, a creature must be capable of being in all, or at least most, of the psychological states that are involved in the identity conditions of that first state.

Now in any normal human being, a psychological state is causally and/or probabilistically linked to an enormous variety of other psychological states. Hence, according to psychofunctionalism, an enormous variety of psychological states are involved in the identity conditions of any psychological state that can be exemplified in a normal human being. Unfortunately, it seems to follow that if an organism is considerably less complicated than a normal human being, the psychological states of a normal human being are forever outside its range. Thus, where ψ is any psychological state and S is the set of psychological states to which ψ is linked in human beings, it is typically the case that less complicated organisms are incapable of being in more than a handful of the members of S.

Consider pain. In normal human beings, pain has a tendency to cause aversion, anxiety, the desire to obtain an analgesic, the desire to escape from a traumatic stimulus, the desire to solicit help from others, and beliefs to the effect that one's body has been damaged or is undergoing a stressful adaptive process. It also has a tendency to cause us to recall past pains, to compare pains with one another, to worry about future pains, to curse pain, to wonder about justice in the cosmos, and to feel sympathetic concern for others when they are suffering from pains of their own. These tendencies are partially constitutive of the role that pain plays in the normal human being. In view of this, it seems reasonable to say that pain plays a different role in normal human beings than it does in normal raccoons and normal gophers. It is probably true that raccoons can experience aversion and anxiety, and also that they can desire to escape from traumatic stimuli. But it seems most unlikely that the other states on our list are within a raccoon's ken. And the same is true of gophers. Does it seem at all likely that gophers wonder about cosmic justice?

There are three ways of responding to this objection that must be considered.

The first response asserts that there is an inconsistency between a proposition that figures prominently in the second absent qualia argument and one of the propositions that is presupposed by the present objection. In expounding the second absent qualia argument, I claimed that we are unwilling to attribute sensations to beings that are radically different from ourselves (for example, to silicon-based androids). Here, however, I have presupposed that beings as different from ourselves as raccoons and gophers are capable of experiencing pain. Isn't the foregoing claim inconsistent with this presupposition? At the very least, shouldn't we say that there is a certain amount of tension between them?

I cannot address this response in this chapter, but I will argue in Chapter 9 that there are considerations that show that it is entirely appropriate for us to attribute sensations to raccoons and gophers, and to members of other biological species that are not too distant from our own. These considerations vindicate the second heterogeneity argument. However, as it turns out, they have no tendency to show that it would be appropriate to attribute sensations to silicon-based androids.

So they have no tendency to undermine the second absent qualia argument.

The second response seeks to block the objection by appealing to functional properties that involve a very limited range of internal states. According to this response, although it is true that pain does not have the same effects in simpler organisms as it does in human beings, it is also true that its effects in simpler organisms are a subset of its effects in us. Thus, the response continues, even if raccoons and gophers are not known for their tendency to reflect on cosmic justice, it is at least true – and it is acknowledged by the objection to be true – that they can feel aversion and anxiety, and can desire to escape from traumatic stimuli. But it follows that there is a functional property – albeit an extremely simple one, involving only a handful of interconnections between internal states – that is common to the pains of human beings and to the pains of these lesser creatures. Psychofunctionalists can identify *being in a pain* with this simple functional property.

There are two problems with this response. First, it is probably false that pain is coextensive – even in normal human beings – with any simple functional property. Certainly it is not coextensive with one that involves no psychological states other than aversion, anxiety, and the desire to escape. There are certain types of pain that have no tendency to make one anxious, and that have no tendency to make one want to escape. Equally, there are sensations that have both of these tendencies, and a tendency to cause aversion as well, but that fail to count as types of pain. Second, from the point of view of psychofunctionalism, it is wrong to think that a raccoon or a gopher can be in states that count as aversion, anxiety, and the desire to escape. For psychofunctionalists are committed to saying that these states are individuated in part by their relations to other psychological states, and it is clear that the states in question are linked in normal human beings to an enormous range of other psychological states. The most that a psychofunctionalist can say is that raccoons and gophers are capable of being in states that are functionally similar to aversion, anxiety, and the desire to escape. But this is not enough for the psychofunctionalist's purposes. The psychofunctionalist must at all costs avoid identifying pain with a disjunction of functional properties that are similar to one another. Psychofunctionalists claim that pain is a functional kind, not that it is a disjunction of functional kinds. (Of course, if psychofunctionalists were permitted to appeal to disjunctions of functional properties in responding to the second heterogeneity argument, it would be necessary to allow type materialists to appeal to disjunctions of physical properties in responding to the functionalists' objections to their position.)

The third response is an attempt to show that the second response is more viable than it at first appears. Specifically, it addresses the objection we have just been considering: the objection that, because psychofunctionalism implies that the effects of pain are individuated by *their* effects, psychofunctionalists are not in a position to claim that the effects of pain in lower animals are a subset of their effects in human beings. The third response argues that this objection can be circumvented.

The key idea of the third response is the notion of a *core component* of the functional role of a mental state. What is intended here can best be explained in terms of examples. There is a clear difference between such effects of pain as aversion, anxiety, and the desire to escape, on the one hand, and such effects as cursing and wondering about cosmic justice, on the other. The former effects are more fundamental than the latter. In view of this difference, it seems appropriate to say that the tendency to cause aversion, the tendency to cause anxiety, and the tendency to cause the desire to escape are more central to the functional role of pain than are the tendency to cause cursing and the tendency to cause musings about cosmic justice. We can express this centrality by saying that the first three tendencies are core components of the functional role of pain.

We need to use the notion of a core component in discussing the functional roles of other mental states. Consider the desire to escape. In concert with beliefs it can cause one to move rapidly away from a harmful stimulus, and it can also cause one to say, "It's time to move on." It is clearly true that the former effect is more fundamental than the latter. By the same token, it is clear that the tendency to cause the former effect is more central to the functional role of the desire to escape than is the tendency to cause the latter effect. Again, we can express this centrality by saying that the tendency to move away from a stimulus is a core component of the causal role of the desire to escape.

So much for preliminaries. The point of the third response can now be formulated as follows: Even though pain has different effects in raccoons and gophers than in human beings, it is nonetheless true that the core components of the causal role of pain are the same in all three cases. But then, setting aside any other problems that may confront the functionalist project, we can say that there is an adequate basis for a functionalist account of pain; for we can say that pain is identical with the functional property that corresponds to the core of the functional role of pain.

The main problem with this third response is that the notion of a core component is not one that the functionalist is entitled to use. The notion of a core component was explained in terms of the notion of a fundamental effect. And to say that certain of the effects of pain are more fundamental than others is to say, I think, that it is the *biological function* of pain to produce the former effects. (I am here using "biological function" with the sense it has in such statements as "It is the biological function of the epiglottis to keep food out of the windpipe" and "It is the biological function of heartbeats to cause the blood to circulate.") Assuming that this is correct, the third response commits the functionalist to holding that it is necessary to use the notion of a biological function in explaining the notion of a functional role, and also in picking out the functional roles of individual sensory states. But if it is necessary to use the notion of a biological function in explaining the notion of a functional role, then the internal states of nonbiological androids cannot be said to occupy functional roles in the same sense in which this can be said of the internal states of organisms. Accordingly, it seems that the third response commits functionalists to abandoning one of their most cherished goals – that of providing an account of sensory states that makes it possible for us to see nonbiological beings as sharing such states.

5. My fifth objection to psychofunctionalism is a counterpart of the third objection to analytic functionalism. It might be called the *second epistemological argument.*

A few preliminary remarks. Let S be a normal human being and let x be any pain that belongs to S. According to psychofunctionalism, x has two properties that are highly germane to the fact that it is a pain. One is an intrinsic property. It is the state-type that plays the role that is characteristic of pain in S. The other one is a functional property – the functional property that is associated with the given functional role. Let us call the first of these properties "Jones" and the other one "Smith." In what does the alleged germaneness of these two properties to the fact that x is a pain consist? According to psychofunctionalism, Jones is germane because it plays the role that is characteristic of pain, and because x's having a property that plays this role is what makes it possible for x to have Smith – the functional property. And, again according to psychofunctionalism, Smith is germane because the property *being a pain* is identical with it.

It follows, of course, that if psychofunctionalism is correct, then, when one believes that one of one's sensations is a pain, one is in effect believing that the sensation in question is an instance of Smith. It seems, however, that this consequence of psychofunctionalism must be wrong, for it seems that the consequence is incompatible with certain of our intuitions about what it is that justifies us in making first-person ascriptions of pain. Thus, it seems that we have an intuition that indicates that it cannot be Smith that provides our justification for making such ascriptions. Equally, it seems that we have a second intuition to the effect that, because it isn't Smith that provides our justification, Smith cannot be the property that is ascribed.

The first intuition may be formulated as follows: Whether one is justified in believing that one of one's sensations is a pain depends only on whether the sensation presents a certain intrinsic nature to introspection. It is not necessary to be aware of any relational facts involving the sensation. If one is introspectively aware of the sensation as having a certain intrinsic characteristic, one is justified in believing that it is a pain. Period.

It follows immediately from this first intuition that Smith does not provide our justification for first-person ascriptions of pain. For Smith is not an intrinsic characteristic. (No sensation can exemplify Smith simply by virtue of having a particular intrinsic nature. Rather, if a sensation exemplifies Smith, it must stand in certain relation to other things, including things that are inaccessible to introspection.) By the same token, assuming that it is either Jones or Smith that provides the justification for first-person ascriptions, it follows immediately that the justification comes from Jones.

The second intuition can be expressed by saying that pains are self-presenting. There are various ways of spelling this intuition out. Thus, it can be spelled out by saying that there is no gap between appearance and reality in the case of pain – that the entity that presents a pain to introspection is identical with the entity that is thereby presented. The intuition can also be expressed by saying that the fact that justifies one in believing that a sensation is a pain is identical with the fact that makes the belief in question true.

Because we have already seen that it isn't Smith that provides our justification for first-person ascriptions of pain, this second intuition forces us to conclude that it isn't Smith that determines whether such ascriptions are true. That is to say, if a subject has a true first-person belief to the effect that a given sensation is a pain, then, although it may well be the case that the sensation in question exemplifies Smith, it can't be the fact that it exemplifies Smith that makes the belief true. The belief must be made true by some other fact involving the sensation. (Assuming that it is Jones that provides our justification for first-person ascriptions, the second intuition implies that our subject's belief is made true by the fact that the sensation exemplifies Jones.)

It follows that psychofunctionalism is mistaken. No matter what metaphysical position about sensations we may wish to take, we must preserve the semantic intuition that *being a pain* is the characteristic that confers truth on ascriptions of pain. Because we have found that it cannot be Smith that confers truth on such ascriptions, we are obliged by this semantic intuition to deny that Smith is identical with *being a pain*.

There is reason to believe that the two intuitions about justification are widely shared. To be sure, there are philosophers who view one or both of the intuitions with suspicion. However, it may be that their suspicions will be at least partially allayed by the theory of introspective awareness of sensations that is presented in Part Three. The theory in question is largely inspired by the intuitions. Hence, if the theory is successful, it may reasonably be thought to provide the intuitions with support, or even with a full vindication.

4

In defense of type materialism

If the arguments up to this point have been successful, we have reason to hope that type materialism is correct. We have encountered arguments that purport to show that type materialism is superior to dualism and the double-aspect theory, and also some arguments that purport to show that functionalism is badly flawed. In view of these arguments, it looks as though the only alternatives to accepting type materialism are (1) to deny the existence of our subject matter (that is, to reject the realist attitude toward sensations that we have assumed from the start), and (2) to accept the nihilistic view that sensations exist but are too elusive to be caught in the net of any metaphysical theory. Although there are people who favor (1) or (2), most of us would be deeply distressed if we were forced to embrace one of them.

Still, it would be premature to infer that type materialism is true; for there are a number of objections against it, and some of these objections have a certain amount of prima facie appeal. Indeed, there are objections against it that are widely thought to be conclusive.

The objections are of three kinds. First, there are arguments that dualists have constructed with a view to showing that their position is to be preferred to token materialism. Type materialism implies token materialism, and it is therefore at risk from all of the arguments that are directed against the latter. Second, there are arguments that concede that token materialism may be true, but that seek to show that any stronger form of materialism must be wrong. And third, there are arguments that attempt to discredit the realist attitude toward sensations that type materialism presupposes. The members of this third group are directed primarily against the *concept* of a sensation. If a

Some of the material in this chapter is excerpted from my paper "In Defense of Type Materialism," *Synthese* 59 (1984), 295–320. I have been helped considerably by conversations and/or correspondence with Ivan Fox, Allan Hazen, Henry Jacoby, Robert Kirk, William G. Lycan, R.J. Nelson, Sydney Shoemaker, G. Lynn Stephens, Willem de Vries, and Stephen White.

83

concept suffers from a deep internal incoherence of some sort, or it is impossibly vague, or it carries a number of constitutive presuppositions that are sharply at variance with the facts, then, presumably, it must be set aside. The arguments in question purport to show that the concept of a sensation has one or more of these flaws.

Over the centuries the enemies of type materialism have been quite busy, and it is therefore impossible to discuss all of the objections they have raised. I will have to choose a sample from each of the three categories. In general, I will select the strongest arguments that each category has to offer. However, I will also include several arguments that seem to me to be comparatively weak – the reason being that historically they have been quite influential. I will discuss members of the first category in sections I–III, members of the second in sections IV–VII, and members of the third in sections VIII–IX.

I

There is a family of pro-dualist arguments that seek to exploit the intuition that sensory states are better known than physical states. Many of these *epistemological arguments* are quite venerable, being implicit in the writings of Descartes and perhaps even in earlier writings.

One member of the family opens with the claim that it is possible to be absolutely certain as to whether one has a sensation of a certain type, and then contrasts this certainty with the epistemic status of our beliefs about physical occurrences in the brain. Kurt Baier gives expression to this line of thought with engaging vivacity in the following passage:

> To say that one day our physiological knowledge will increase to such an extent that we shall be able to make absolutely reliable encephalograph-based claims about people's experiences, is only to say that, if carefully checked, our encephalograph-based claims about 'experiences' will always be *correct*, i.e. will make the *same claims* as a *truthful* introspective report. If correct encephalograph-based claims about Smith's experiences contradict Smith's introspective reports, we shall be entitled to infer that he is lying. In that sense, what Smith says will no longer go. But we cannot of course infer that he is making a mistake, for that is nonsense. . . . However good the evidence may be, such a physiological theory can never be used to show to the sufferer that he was mistaken in thinking that he had a pain, for such a mistake is inconceivable. The sufferer's epistemological authority must therefore be better than the best physiological

theory can ever be. Physiology can therefore never provide a person with more than *evidence* that someone else is having an experience of one sort or another. It can never lay down *criteria* for saying that someone is having an experience of a certain sort. Talk about brain-processes therefore must be about something other than talk about experiences. Hence, introspective reports and brain-process talk cannot be merely different ways of talking about the same thing.[1]

Although there is a lot going on in this passage, it seems fair to say that Baier's central idea can be captured in a formal argument that looks something like this:

> **First premise.** Sensations can be known to exist with certainty.
>
> **Second premise.** Brain processes cannot be known to exist with certainty.
>
> **Third premise.** (Leibniz's law). If x has a property that y fails to have, then x is not identical with y.
>
> **Conclusion.** Sensations are not identical with brain processes.

Now it is possible to attack this argument by criticizing the first premise; for, as we will see later on, there are grounds for doubting the traditional view that beliefs about sensations are incorrigible. However, to proceed in this way is to succumb to tunnel vision. Even if we cannot be absolutely certain of the existence and nature of our sensations, it is surely true that knowledge of sensations is superior in *some* ways to knowledge of physical states. For one thing, it seems that one's epistemic contact with the sensory realm has a higher degree of immediacy than one's contact with the physical world.

Fortunately, it is possible to discredit a large subclass of the class of epistemological arguments by pointing out that it is fallacious to combine Leibniz's law with sentences containing verbs of propositional attitude – that is, with sentences that are concerned with psychological states like certainty, knowledge, and belief. Consider the following argument:

> **First premise.** Little Sally is certain that the sum of 1 and 2 is 3.
>
> **Second premise.** Little Sally is not certain that the cube root of 27 is 3.

---

1 Kurt Baier, "Smart on Sensations," *Australasian Journal of Philosophy* 40 (1962), 57–68. The quoted passage appears on pp. 64–65.

Third premise. If x has a property that y fails to have, then x is not identical with y.

Conclusion. 3 is not identical with the cube root of 27.

The premises of this argument are true, and the conclusion is manifestly false. Hence, because it is similar in form to the preceding argument, it shows that the latter is fallacious. Moreover, this is just the beginning of the story. It is easy to construct similar arguments to show that it is fallacious to combine Leibniz's law with sentences containing "knows that," "is aware that," "has evidence that," and "believes that." A fortiori, it can be shown that it is fallacious to combine Leibniz's law with sentences containing "knows with immediacy that," "has conclusive evidence that," "is directly aware that," and other expressions of the same sort.

It would, however, be a mistake to think that all epistemological arguments misuse Leibniz's law in this way. There are members of this class that eschew verbs of propositional attitude. Here is a typical example:

First premise. It is possible to be directly aware of one's sensations.

Second premise. It isn't possible to be directly aware of physical occurrences.

Third premise. If x has a property that y fails to have, then x is not identical with y.

Conclusion. Sensations are not identical with physical occurrences.

The premises of this argument seem correct: Sensory states are self-presenting, but awareness of physical occurrences depends on the mediation of internal phenomena that are caused by the occurrences and that serve to represent them. Moreover, even though "aware" stands for a propositional attitude when it occurs as a component of the construction "aware that," its sense in "aware of" is different. Instead of standing for a relation between minds and propositions, it stands for a relation between minds and concrete substances or concrete events. When used with this second sense, its interactions with Leibniz's law are entirely innocent.

Still, there is a fatal flaw: The second premise begs the question. To be sure, it is true in most cases that awareness of physical occurrences has to be mediated by internal representations that are distinct from the occurrences themselves. But what if sensations are identical with a subset of the set of physical occurrences? If this is the case, then there is a set of physical occurrences that are – albeit without one's knowing it – exceptions to the second premise. Thus, it appears that it is necessary to show that materialism is false before one can be in a position to claim that the second premise is true.

II

In a widely discussed essay, Thomas Nagel points out that a neurophysiological account of the brain must inevitably fail to tell us *what it is like* to have a sensation of a particular kind.[2] It follows, he claims, that materialism is incapable of capturing the qualitative aspects of experience. Nagel does not represent himself as a dualist, but it is nonetheless true that his argument questions the validity (and even the intelligibility) of token materialism. Accordingly, the argument belongs to our first category.

Setting questions of interpretation aside for a moment, and sticking as closely as possible to Nagel's actual words, the argument can be summarized as follows:

> **First premise.** It is impossible to know what it is like to have the sensations that another creature has unless one is capable of taking the point of view of that creature.

> **Second premise.** It is possible to know all of the physical facts about a creature without taking the point of view of that creature.

> **Conclusion.** There is an obstacle to providing a physicalist reduction of sensations that may turn out to be insuperable.

Even a deeply committed materialist will perforce feel that this argument has a certain allure. Nevertheless, it is clear that, as it stands, the argument leaves a great deal to be desired: It contains several concepts that are highly problematical, and it falls quite a bit short of formal validity. The question therefore arises whether it is possible to find a similar argument that can be seen to incorporate Nagel's premises and that meets appropriate standards of clarity, organization, and rigor. Unless such an argument can be found, it seems fair to set Nagel's

2 Thomas Nagel, "What Is It Like to Be a Bat?" *The Philosophical Review* LXXXIII (1974), 435–50.

original argument aside, and to take the view that its allure is a kind of logical mirage.

In what has come to be the standard response to the argument, it is maintained that any attempt to upgrade it is doomed to failure. Specifically, it is maintained that one will either use Leibniz's law in a fallacious way or wind up begging the question.[3] Thus, commentators generally suggest that one will wind up with an argument that belongs to the same family as one of these:

(A) **First premise.** It is impossible to form adequate concepts of the sensations of another creature unless one is capable of taking the point of view of that creature.

Second premise. It is fully possible to form adequate concepts of the physical states of another creature even if one is altogether incapable of taking the point of view of that creature.

Third premise. If x has a property that y fails to have, then x is not identical with y.

Conclusion. Sensations are not identical with physical states.

(B) **First premise.** The sensations of one creature cannot be known by another creature unless the second creature is capable of taking the point of view of the first.

Second premise. The physical states of one creature can be known by another creature even if the second creature is altogether incapable of taking the point of view of the first.

Third premise. If x has a property that y fails to have, x is not identical with y.

Conclusion. Sensations are not identical with physical states.

It is clear that these arguments are fallacious. As for (A), although it is true that the expression "concept of" does not stand for a propositional attitude, its sense is closely related to the senses of terms for propositional attitudes, and as a result, all bets are off when it is combined with Leibniz's law. This can be seen by reflecting on the following example:

3 As far as I know, I was the first to take this line. See my "Of Bats, Brains, and Minds," *Philosophy and Phenomenological Research* XXXVIII (1977), 100–106. A more recent (and more convincing) elaboration of this position may be found in Paul Churchland, "Reduction, Qualia, and the Direct Introspection of Brain States," *The Journal of Philosophy* LXXXII (1985), 8–28.

First premise. Little Sally has an adequate concept of heat.

Second premise. Little Sally does not have an adequate concept of molecular kinetic energy.

Third premise. If x has a property that y fails to have, then x is not identical with y.

Conclusion. Heat is not identical with molecular kinetic energy.

Here we have true premises and a false conclusion; so the argument must be fallacious. As for (B), although it might at first seem to commit the same fallacy, it turns out that this perception is inaccurate. Like "aware," "know" has a sense in which its logical properties are quite different than the ones it has when it appears in conjunction with "that." (This is the sense of "know" that we find in "Alas, poor Yorick! I knew him, Horatio.") However, (B) begs the question in much the same way as the last argument in the previous section. Thus, on the assumption that we materialists are right in holding that sensations are identical with physical states, the first premise of (B) is false. For materialism implies that we can gain knowledge of the sensations of another creature – albeit without knowing *that* we are gaining such knowledge – by coming to know the creature's physical states.

Although I feel that this response makes contact with some of the undercurrents of thought that account for the appeal of Nagel's argument, I also feel that it misses the main point. As I see it, it is impossible to do full justice to the first premise of the argument unless one acknowledges that its key component – the expression "know what it is like" – is an idiom. It has a complex sense that does not derive directly from the senses of its constituents – a sense that transcends the sense of "concept of" and also the sense of "know" (whether "know" is used as a term for a propositional attitude or is used with the significance it has in "poor Yorick" contexts). Specifically, when one says "x knows what it is like to be a ϕ," one means, at least in part, that x has had experiences of the sort that characteristically accompany being a ϕ. And when one says that "x knows what it is like to have an experience of type ψ," one means, at least in part, that x has had experiences of type ψ. Thus, when Nagel says "Human beings cannot know what it is like to be a bat," he means, at least in part, that we are incapable of having sensations that are similar to those of a bat. And when he says "Human beings cannot know what it is like to have the sensations that accompany sonar perception in bats," he means, at least in part, that we are incapable of having sensations that are similar to sonar-linked sensations. It is clear that these contentions of Nagel's are true! Moreover, it is clear that their relevance is not acknowledged by the standard response to Nagel's argument.

It appears, however, that these reflections simply lead us from the frying pan into the fire: They immunize the argument against the standard response, but in doing so they expose it to an objection that is no less serious. If it is true that "knows" is put to an idiomatic use in the first premise, then its logical role in that premise is quite different from its logical role in the second premise. For in the second premise, "know" has one of its standard senses – either the propositional attitude sense or the "poor Yorick" sense. But this means that the argument involves a fallacy of equivocation.

III

As the reader may recall, in the Introduction we took note of an argument for dualism that runs as follows:

> **First premise.** Conceivability is an adequate test for logical possibility. That is to say, if we can clearly and distinctly conceive of its being the case that p, then it is logically possible for it to be the case that p.
>
> **Second premise.** Where x is any sensory event and y is any physical event whatsoever, it is possible to conceive clearly and distinctly of a situation in which x is not identical with y.
>
> **Third premise.** If it is logically possible that x is not identical with y, then it is false that x is identical with y.
>
> **Conclusion.** Sensory events are not identical with physical events.

I will call this the *Cartesian argument*.

Turning now to the task of assessing the argument, I will begin by conceding the second premise to the dualist. On any natural sense of "conceive," it is true to say that we can conceive clearly and distinctly of situations in which pains exist but in which they are not accompanied by physical events of any sort, and true to say that we can conceive clearly and distinctly of situations in which physical events exist but in which they are not accompanied by pains. A situation of either of these kinds is a situation in which it fails to be true that pains are identical with physical events.

Further, the third premise can be seen to be true by reflecting on (1):

90

> If x is identical with y, it is logically necessary that x is identical
> with y. $\qquad(1)$

As Kripke and others have pointed out, we have reason to believe that
(1) is true.[4] How could it fail to be? Given that x is the very same thing
as y, if one maintained that there is a logically possible world in which
x fails to be identical with y, one would in effect be saying that there is
a logically possible world in which x fails to be identical with itself.
And this latter claim is absurd. So (1) must be true. But the third
premise follows immediately from (1). Thus, (1) implies that if it is not
logically necessary that x is identical with y, then x is not identical with
y in fact. And to say that it is not logically necessary that x is identical
with y is to say that it is logically possible that x is not identical with y.

Because I will soon be appealing to the third premise myself, I will
supplement this defense of it by responding to an objection that some
might raise against (1). Some might be tempted to reject (1) because it
brings us into conflict with a criterion of logical necessity that has
enjoyed quite a bit of visibility in the writings of philosophers. According to this criterion, a proposition is logically necessary if and only if it
is a member of a class of propositions that consists of the conceptual
truths, the laws of logic, and the laws of mathematics. To see why the
criterion poses a problem, consider (2):

> Samuel Clemens is identical with Mark Twain. $\qquad(2)$

(2) is not a member of the class consisting of the conceptual truths, the
laws of logic, and the laws of mathematics. Hence, according to the
traditional criterion of logical necessity, it isn't logically necessary that
Samuel Clemens is identical with Mark Twain. However, when (2) is
combined with (1), we get the result that it *is* logically necessary that
Clemens is identical with Twain.

I think this problem shows that we need to revise the familiar
criterion of logical necessity. It will help to introduce a couple of
technical concepts. First, where T_1 and T_2 are terms (that is, either
singular terms or general terms), T_1 may be said to be *necessarily
coreferential* with T_2 if and only if T_1 has the same reference (extension)
as T_2 at every possible world. And second, where P_1 and P_2 are propositions (statements), P_1 may be said to be *strongly equivalent* to P_2 if and only
if P_1 and P_2 satisfy these two conditions: (a) P_1 and P_2 have the same

---

4 See Saul A. Kripke, "Identity and Necessity," in Milton K. Munitz (ed.), *Identity and
Individuation* (New York: New York University Press, 1971), 135–64.

logical form except perhaps at the level of nonlogical terms (that is, a nonlogical term in one proposition might have a higher degree of logical complexity than the corresponding term in the other proposition); and (b) where T_1 and T_2 are terms (singular terms or general terms) that occupy corresponding positions in P_1 and P_2, T_1 is necessarily coreferential with T_2. I can now formulate a revised version of the foregoing criterion. Instead of saying that a proposition is logically necessary if and only if it is a member of the class consisting of the conceptual truths, the laws of logic, and the laws of mathematics, I suggest that we say that a proposition is logically necessary if and only if either (i) it is a member of this class, or (ii) it is strongly equivalent to a proposition that is a member of the class. Is this proposal well-motivated? Does it seem reasonable to say that propositions that satisfy (ii) are logically necessary? Yes. Let P_1 be a proposition that satisfies (ii). Because P_1 satisfies (ii), there exists a proposition P_2 such that (a) P_2 satisfies (i), and (b) P_1 is strongly equivalent to P_2. It follows from (b) that P_1 is just like P_2 in all logical and semantic properties that play a role in determining truth values in possible worlds. Hence, P_1 and P_2 must have the same truth values in all possible worlds. Surely this is an excellent reason for saying that they have the same modal status. Further, P_2 counts as logically necessary by virtue of satisfying (i) (that is, by virtue of satisfying the original criterion). Hence, assuming that the original criterion is sound, we have an excellent reason for saying that P_1 is logically necessary.[5]

Assuming that the proposal is acceptable, we can lay the problem of two paragraphs ago to rest. For there is good reason to believe that (2) satisfies condition (ii) in the revised version of the criterion. This can be seen as follows. First, because "x is identical with x" is a law of logic, "Samuel Clemens is identical with Samuel Clemens" is a law of logic too. So it is a member of the class consisting of the conceptual truths, the laws of logic, and the laws of mathematics. So, by (i), "Samuel Clemens is identical with Samuel Clemens" is logically necessary. Second, as Kripke and others have shown, the thesis that a proper name has the same reference at every possible world is strongly supported by

---

5 I am prescinding here from the problems that arise from the fact that identity statements may be truth-valueless in possible worlds in which their constituent singular terms do not refer. The qualifications needed to deal with these problems would not materially affect the point at issue, but they would add substantially to the length and complexity of the exposition.

intuitions about the meanings of names.[6] Assuming that the thesis is true, because "Samuel Clemens" and "Mark Twain" have the same reference at the actual world, these two names must be necessarily co-referential. But then "Samuel Clemens is identical with Samuel Clemens" is strongly equivalent to (2).[7] So, by (ii), (2) is logically necessary.

It appears, then, that the second and third premises of the Cartesian argument are correct. By the same token it appears that the argument stands or falls with the thesis that conceivability is an adequate test for logical possibility. However, this thesis is false. We can appreciate this by continuing to reflect on (2). Can we conceive of a situation in which (2) is false? Of course! Can we clearly and distinctly conceive of such a situation? Of course! Hence, if we were to maintain that conceivability is an adequate test for logical possibility, we would have to conclude that it is possible that Clemens is not identical with Twain. Then, because of the third premise of the Cartesian argument, we would be forced to conclude that it is just plain false that Clemens is identical with Twain. But this conclusion is wrong.

Is it really as clear as I have maintained that it is possible to conceive of a situation in which Clemens is not identical with Twain? In addition to being intuitively plausible, the claim can be defended by an argument.

> **First premise.** The concept of Samuel Clemens is not identical with the concept of Mark Twain, and the concepts are not linked by logical ties of any other kind.
>
> **Second premise.** If the members of a pair of concepts are not linked by logical ties, it is possible to conceive of something as a thing that falls under one of the concepts without conceiving of it as a thing that falls under the other.
>
> **Third premise.** If it is possible to conceive of something as a thing that falls under one member of a pair of concepts without conceiving of it as a thing that falls under the other, it is possible to conceive of something as a thing that falls under one of the concepts and that fails to fall under the other.

6 See Saul A. Kripke, *Naming and Necessity* (Cambridge, MA: Harvard University Press, 1980).
7 See note 5.

> **Conclusion.** It is possible to conceive of a situation in which Samuel Clemens exists and in which Mark Twain does not exist – that is, a situation in which it is false that Samuel Clemens is identical with Mark Twain.

The first premise is a factual claim, but it seems to me to be obviously correct. The second and third premises are partially constitutive of our notion of conceivability. (Because there can be logically independent concepts of Clemens and of Twain which are both highly coherent and highly detailed, we can extend this argument to show that it is possible to conceive clearly and distinctly of a situation in which it is false that Clemens is identical with Twain.)

In sum, there is at least one class of cases in which conceivability fails to be an adequate test for possibility. Specifically, where p is an identity proposition involving two different names (or two different rigid designators of some other sort), we cannot use conceivability to determine whether it is possible that p.[8] When we try to use conceivability as a test in cases of this sort, we reach conclusions that we know to be false. Further, because the Cartesian argument requires an assumption that is incompatible with this finding (at minimum, it requires the assumption that we can use conceivability to determine the modal status of identity propositions of the form "sensation a is identical with brain process b"), it follows that the Cartesian argument is unsound.

Although I reject the view about the relationship between conceivability and possibility that we find in the Cartesian argument, I have no wish to deny that there are cases in which it is legitimate to make use of conceivability in determining the modal status of propositions. On the contrary. Thus, as I indicated in Chapter 3, it seems clear to me that we have every right to test whether a proposition is conceptually true by checking to see whether we can conceive of a situation in which the proposition fails to hold. I also think that we are entitled to make use of

---

8 The notion of a rigid designator is due to Kripke. (See his *Naming and Necessity*, pp. 48–49.) A rigid designator is any term whose reference remains constant from possible world to possible world. Thus, for example, "Benjamin Franklin" is rigid but "the inventor of bifocals" is not: Whereas the former picks Franklin out directly, the latter succeeds in picking him out only by mentioning one of his contingent properties. In addition to including proper names, the class of rigid designators includes names of natural kinds (for example, "gold," "pain"), descriptions that pick things out by mentioning their essential properties (for example, "the substance whose molecules consist of one oxygen atom and two hydrogen atoms"), and tokens of certain demonstratives (for example, tokens of "this house").

conceivability in checking to see whether a proposition is a law of logic. And conceivability may admit of other uses as well.[9]

IV

This brings us to a series of objections that more or less concede that token materialism may be true, but that purport to show that type materialism is wrong. Here, in the words of Jerome Shaffer, is the first member of the series:

> Let us return to the man reporting the red afterimage. He was aware of the occurrence of something or other, of some feature or other. Now it seems to me obvious that he was not necessarily aware of the state of his brain at this time (I doubt that most of us are ever aware of the state of our brain) nor, in general, necessarily aware of any physical features of his body at that time. He might, of course, have been incidentally aware of some physical feature, but not insofar as he was aware of the red afterimage as such. Yet he was definitely aware of something, or else how could he have made that report? So he must have been aware of some nonphysical feature. That is the only way of explaining how he was aware of anything at all.[10]

Armstrong considers essentially the same argument in the course of cataloging the main objections to his position. Thus, he imagines an opponent who argues as follows:

> Central-state materialism holds that when we are *aware* of our mental states what we are aware of are mere physical states of our brain. But we

9 I would like to add, however, that there are cases other than ones involving identity propositions in which conceivability fails to serve as an adequate test. For example, it is clear that we are perfectly capable of conceiving of situations in which the denials of certain mathematical propositions are true, but this seems not to be a good reason to deny that the propositions in question are necessary. (Here I have certain existential propositions primarily in mind – propositions such as "There exists a system of numbers that is closed under the operation of taking square roots.") Again, many philosophers maintain that propositions about the origins of material substances are necessary, and that the same is true of propositions that ascribe sortals to individual substances and events. Assuming that they are right, how do we recognize that these propositions are necessary? One suggestion is that we come to appreciate their necessity by finding that we are incapable of conceiving of situations in which they are false. But this suggestion is wrong. I am quite sure, for example, that we do not come to realize that "Reagan is a person rather than an android" is necessary by finding that we cannot conceive of situations in which Reagan *is* an android. For it is quite clear that we can conceive of such situations.
10 See Jerome Shaffer, *Philosophy of Mind* (Englewood Cliffs, NJ: Prentice-Hall, 1968), p. 46.

95

are certainly not aware of the mental states as states of the brain. What then are we aware of mental states as? Are we not aware of them as states of a quite peculiar, mental, sort?[11]

One also encounters the objection when one hears it said that there is an "unbridgeable gulf" between conscious experiences and brain processes, and when one is told that there is no way of accounting for the "striking qualitative differences" between the essential natures of events of these two kinds. Another manifestation is the claim that, for example, the difference between a red sensation and a sour sensation is self-evidently a *different* difference than the difference between the neural processes that accompany them. Yet another manifestation is the idea that qualitative characteristics differ from neurological characteristics in that the former are self-evidently simple and unanalyzable whereas the latter are analyzable in terms of the properties and relations of microevents. And, less obviously, it underlies the claim that conscious experiences enjoy a "luminosity" or a "phosphorescence" that brain processes lack.

When Shaffer's line of thought is set out as a formal argument, it comes to this:

> **First premise.** When one is introspectively aware of a conscious experience, one is aware of it as having a qualitative characteristic.

> **Second premise.** If qualitative characteristics were identical with neurological characteristics, then when one is aware of an event as an event that has a qualitative characteristic, one would be aware of it as an event that has a neurological characteristic.

> **Third premise.** When one is introspectively aware of a conscious experience, one is not aware of it as an event that has any neurological characteristics.

> **Conclusion.** Qualitative characteristics are not identical with neurological characteristics.

This formulation is too sober and clinical to do justice to the power of the intuitions that give rise to the argument; but in its own way, it captures all of the ideas that play a logically essential role.

In order to reply to this argument, I need a premise about awareness that seems uncontroversial – namely, the view that *to be aware of a*

---

11 David M. Armstrong, *A Materialist Theory of the Mind* (New York: Humanities Press, 1968), p. 78.

particular as a ϕ is to have an experience that leads one to subsume the particular under the concept of a ϕ. Assuming that this view is correct, the second premise of the argument carries the following presupposition: If qualitative characteristics were identical with neurological characteristics, then the experiences that lead us to subsume events under our concepts of qualitative characteristics would partially or entirely coincide with the experiences that lead us to subsume events under our concepts of neurological characteristics. As far as I can tell, there is no reason to believe that this presupposition is true.

It is helpful in this connection to reflect on the differences between the circumstances in which our concepts of qualitative characteristics are formed and the circumstances in which our concepts of neurophysiological characteristics are formed. To this end, let us suppose that *being a pain* satisfies the main quasi-empirical presupposition of type materialism – namely, the presupposition that qualitative characteristics are universally correlated with neurophysiological characteristics. Let us also suppose that *being a case of C-fiber stimulation* is the neurophysiological characteristic that is universally correlated with *being a pain*. And let us take note of the following fact: The concept of pain is formed in response to the experiences that one has by virtue of BEING IN a state of mind that instantiates *being a pain*, and the concept of C-fiber stimulation is formed in response to the experiences one has by virtue of (directly or indirectly) OBSERVING a brain state that instantiates *being a case of C-fiber stimulation*. Type materialism requires one to conceptualize this fact in a way that is not required by other theories. Thus, if type materialism is true, the fact comes to this: The concept of pain is formed in response to the experiences one has by virtue of BEING IN a brain state of a certain sort, and the concept of C-fiber stimulation is formed in response to the experiences one has by virtue of OBSERVING a brain state that is a state of the very same sort. However, even when it is stated in the form that is required by type materialism, the fact shows that there is an enormous difference between the factors that shape the concept of pain and the factors that shape the concept of C-fiber stimulation.

In view of the circumstances in which the concept of pain is formed, we can see that the following proposition must be true: To have an experience that leads one to subsume an event under the concept of pain is simply *to have a pain.* That is to say, to have an experience that leads one to subsume an event under the concept of pain is to have an experience that *itself falls under the concept of pain.* Further, in view of the circumstances in which the concept of C-fiber stimulation is acquired, we can see that this second proposition must be true: To have an experience that leads one to subsume an event under the concept of C-fiber stimulation is to have an experience that is produced by using one's sensory apparatus (supplemented or unsupplemented) to *observe* a state of the brain. Now the question is this: Should type materialism encourage us to expect that experiences of the first sort (experiences that fall under the concept of pain) will either partially or fully coincide with experiences of the second sort (experiences produced by using one of the senses to observe the brain)? It is clear, I think, that the answer is "No."[12]

V

In the course of an illuminating critical examination of recent work on the mind–body problem, Stephen White sketches a line of thought that he calls the *property dualism argument*. Here is what he says:

> We are assuming, for simplicity, that a person's qualitative state of pain at *t*, say Smith's, is identical with a physical state, say Smith's brain state X at *t*. Even if this is the case, however, not only do the sense of the expression 'Smith's pain at *t*' and the sense of the expression 'Smith's brain state X at *t*' differ, but the fact that they are coreferential cannot be established on a priori grounds. Thus there must be different properties of Smith's pain (i.e., Smith's brain state X) in virtue of which it is the referent of both terms. In the case of the expressions 'the morning star' and 'the evening star', it is in virtue of the property of being the last heavenly body visible in the morning that Venus is the referent of the first expression. And (since 'the evening star' is not coreferential a priori with 'the morning star') it is in virtue of the *logically distinct* property of being the first heavenly body visible in the evening that it is the referent to the second. The general principle is that if two expressions refer to the same object, and this fact cannot be established a priori, they do so in virtue of different modes of presentation of that referent. These modes of presentation of the object fall on the object's side of the language/world dichotomy. In other words they are aspects of the object in virtue of which our conceptual apparatus picks the object out; they are not aspects of that conceptual apparatus itself. Hence the natural candidates for these modes

---

12 My objection to the Shaffer–Armstrong argument appears to be closely related to the objection that William G. Lycan is expressing when he accuses dualists of having committed the "stereoscopic fallacy." See Lycan's *Consciousness* (Cambridge, MA: M.I.T. Press, 1987), pp. 76–77.

98

of presentation are properties. . . . Since there is no physicalistic description one could plausibly suppose is coreferential a priori with an expression like 'Smith's pain at *t*', no physical property of a pain (i.e., a brain
state of type *X*) could provide the route by which it was picked out by
such an expression. . . .

This argument, which I shall call the *property dualism argument*, shows
that unless there are topic neutral expressions with which mentalistic
descriptions of particular pains are coreferential a priori, we are forced to
acknowledge the existence of mental properties.[13]

By "mental properties" White means *irreducibly* mental properties.
The core of White's argument can be reformulated as follows:

> **First premise.** Where *x* and *y* are any two singular terms, if you can't see
> a priori that *x* is coreferential with *y*, the mode of presentation that is
> associated with *x* must be distinct from the mode of presentation that is
> associated with *y*.
>
> **Second premise.** Modes of presentation are properties – specifically, they
> are properties of the entities they present.
>
> **Lemma.** If the property that is the mode of presentation associated with
> "Smith's pain at *t*" is identical with the property that is the mode of
> presentation associated with some physicalistic description, it is possible
> to see a priori that "Smith's pain at *t*" is coreferential with some physical-
> istic description.
>
> **Third premise.** No physicalistic description is coreferential a priori with
> "Smith's pain at *t*."
>
> **Conclusion.** The property that is the mode of presentation associated
> with "Smith's pain at *t*" is not identical with any property that is
> associated with some physicalistic description (as a mode of presentation).

White then goes on to use this conclusion as a lemma for the following
claim: Unless the property that is the mode of presentation associated
with "Smith's pain at *t*" can be fully captured by a topic neutral
description (that is, unless the property in question is a causal or
functional property of some kind), we will be forced to say that it is an
irreducibly mental property, and by the same token, we will be forced
to recognize that irreducibly mental properties exist.

Why exactly does this line of thought make trouble for type materialism? As I see it, *being a pain* is the property that is the mode of

---

13 Stephen L. White, "Curse of the Qualia," *Synthese* 68 (1986), 333–68. The quoted
material is excerpted from pp. 351–53.

presentation associated with "Smith's pain at t." (At least, it is the mode of presentation associated with this description if we think of the description as one that is being used to make a first-person report.) But if *being a pain* is the mode of presentation associated with "Smith's pain at t," the conclusion of White's main lemma implies that *being a pain* is not identical with any property that is associated with some physicalistic description as a mode of presentation. And it can seem that this implies that *being a pain* is not identical with any physical property.

Fortunately, I think we can see that, despite appearances to the contrary, type materialism can withstand this line of thought. This is because, despite appearances to the contrary, White's lemma cannot be used to show that the mode of presentation associated with "Smith's pain at t" is not identical with any physical property. I do not mean to claim that the lemma is unsound; in my view, White succeeds in showing that the mode of presentation associated with "Smith's pain at t" is not identical with any property that is associated (as a mode of presentation) with a physicalistic description. The point is rather that, despite appearances to the contrary, this conclusion is too weak a claim to undermine type materialism.

Consider the description of "Smith's brain state of type X at t." The property dualism argument tells us that the mode of presentation associated with "Smith's pain at t" is not identical with the mode of presentation associated with this physicalistic description. But what exactly is the mode of presentation with which the latter description is associated? Evidently, it is a property that guides us in recognizing events as members of the extension of "brain state of type X." Thus, it must be the property *looking like such and such when seen through the cerebroscope*, or the property *causing the electroencephalograph to inscribe a curve of such and such shape*, or some other property of the same sort. It is not the property *being a brain state of type X*; for although this property may be said to guide us in recognizing events that belong to the extension of "brain state of type X," the guidance that it provides is entirely indirect. Direct guidance has to come from properties to which our senses are more immediately attuned.

In other words, "Smith's brain state of type X at t" is associated with properties of two kinds. It is associated with the purely neurological property *being a brain state of type X*, and it is associated with a range of properties that brain events have by virtue of their actual and/or potential effects on human sense organs and on laboratory apparatus. Because it is only properties of the second sort that are capable of guiding us directly in using "Smith's brain state of type X at t," it must be a property of the latter sort that is the mode of presentation associated with this description. Now, if it shows anything about properties at all, the property dualism argument shows only that the property that is the mode of presentation associated with "Smith's pain at t" is not identical with the property that is the mode of presentation associated with "Smith's brain state of type X at t." Thus, the argument shows only that the property that is the mode of presentation associated with "Smith's pain at t" is not identical with a property of the second kind. It has no tendency to show that the former property is not identical with *being a brain state of type X*. By the same token, it has no tendency to count against type materialism.[14]

VI

The next objection is known as the *multiple realization argument*:

> **First premise.** It is nomologically possible for there to be individuals (hereafter called "aliens") that satisfy these three conditions: (1) they have the same behavioral capacities and tendencies as human beings; (2) they have an internal device for collecting, processing, and transmitting information that is functionally isomorphic to the human nervous system; and (3) they have no internal states that can be said to possess neurological characteristics. (The states of the internal computing device are composed of microstates that differ both in structure and in type of matter from the corresponding states of human beings.)
>
> **Second premise.** Aliens enjoy conscious experiences with the same qualitative characteristics as human beings, and their experiences are connected with behavior by the same laws as obtain in the human case.
>
> **Conclusion.** Qualitative characteristics are not identical with neurological characteristics.

This argument has enjoyed wide currency in the literature.

I propose to focus here on the second premise. In effect, we have already found reason to doubt that the functionalist has a right to claim that this premise is true. Thus, in Chapter 3, we noticed in effect that it is a mistake to suppose that we are justified in ascribing sensations to aliens. However, I would like to supplement the foregoing discussion

---

14 A similar line of thought is developed by Richard N. Boyd in his "Materialism Without Reduction," in Ned Block (ed.), *Readings in the Philosophy of Psychology*, Vol. I (Cambridge, MA: Harvard University Press, 1980), 67–106. See especially pp. 83–85.

by replying to a line of thought that a functionalist might use to defend the multiple realization argument. The line of thought I have in mind goes like this: The hypothesis that aliens have experiences with the same qualitative characteristics as ours provides the best explanation of their behavior; hence, in view of the best explanation principle, we are justified in concluding that the hypothesis is true. This argument appears prima facie to be quite strong.

On closer inspection, however, it turns out that we are not in a position to apply the best explanation principle in the present context. For it is possible to account for alien behavior by another hypothesis, and there is no reason to think that this other hypothesis is inferior to the hypothesis that aliens have internal states with qualitative characteristics. According to the second hypothesis, the internal states of aliens lack qualitative characteristics, but they have characteristics that play roles in the mental lives of aliens that are similar to the roles played by qualitative characteristics in our mental lives. Thus, whereas the first hypothesis can be seen as the claim that aliens satisfy the totality of psychological laws that human beings satisfy, including the laws that refer to qualitative characteristics, the second hypothesis can be seen as the claim that alien psychological laws can be obtained from domestic laws by reinterpreting all predicates that denote qualitative characteristics over a set of properties that (1) are instantiated by the internal states of aliens, and (2) are functionally equivalent to the properties that the predicates normally express.

It follows trivially from this description of the second hypothesis that the two hypotheses are equivalent in explanatory power. The first hypothesis provides an explanation of a pattern of alien behavior if and only if the second hypothesis provides an isomorphic explanation. However, it might be thought that the first hypothesis should be preferred to the second on the grounds of simplicity. After all, the second hypothesis calls for a duplication of psychological laws, thereby complicating our overall theory, and it might be thought that the duplication is unnecessary. Further, it is often held that there is a methodological principle that counsels conservatism. Because the second hypothesis calls for a change in our overall theory that can seem to be gratuitous, it might be thought that this methodological principle calls the second hypothesis into question.

These complaints about the second hypothesis would be legitimate if it were true that the explananda that come to the fore when we focus on alien behavior are identical to the explananda that come to the fore when we focus on human behavior. But in fact the explananda are different, and the foregoing appeals to simplicity and conservatism are invalidated by their differences. The explananda are different because human behavior is only identical to alien behavior up to an isomorphism. To see this, consider a case in which someone withdraws his or her hand from a hot stove, and in which we explain the motion of the hand by referring to a pain. Here the explanandum is the motion of a *human hand*, where a human hand is conceived as something that is a member of a certain natural kind. No such explanandum comes to the fore when we consider aliens. To be sure, it is possible to say that aliens have hands; but when we say this, we are using "hand" in a new and extended sense. Alien hands do not belong to the same natural kind as human hands. Indeed, unlike the paw of a dog, an alien hand does not even belong to a neighboring kind. For it is an essential feature of a human hand and of a dog's paw that they contain nerves, but nerves are entirely foreign to alien hands. Thus, when we use "hand" in talking about alien appendages, either it stands for a different kind than it does when we talk about human hands, or our use of it is temporarily guided by a criterion of what is to count as a hand that is purely functional.

Up to this point it has been assumed that aliens have no neural tissue whatsoever. Let us now suppose instead that aliens have nerves at their peripheries, and that they differ from us only in having central computing devices that are devoid of neurological qualities. (We might suppose that aliens of this sort are created by replacing the brains of certain human beings with artificial brains, and by equipping the latter with some means of communicating with peripheral nerves.) Under this new assumption, alien behavioral explananda are type-identical with domestic behavioral explananda. However, the totality of alien explananda still differs considerably from the totality of all domestic explananda, for the former totality includes central explananda that are quite different than all of the explananda in the latter totality. To see this, notice that it is reasonable to accept the following pair of propositions: First, there are causal relations between qualitative events and human brain processes; and second, these causal relations mediate many of the causal relations between qualitative events and human behavioral events. Assuming that the two propositions are correct, if a hypothesis claims that the aetiology of alien behavior is isomorphic to the aetiology of human behavior, it must explain some of the events that take place in alien central computing devices in terms either of qualitative events or counterparts of qualitative events. Because all events that take place in alien central computing devices belong to different kinds than human brain processes, neither simplicity nor conservatism can require us to explain the former events in the same way that we explain the latter. And this means that neither simplicity nor conservatism can require us to explain the former events in terms of qualitative events instead of explaining them in terms of counterparts of qualitative events.

Simplicity and conservatism may require us to explain similar phenomena (that is, phenomena that belong to the same kind) in similar ways, but they do not require us to explain different phenomena in similar ways. Thus, appeals to simplicity and conservatism are inappropriate in the present context. We cannot use them to establish the claim that the first hypothesis is superior to the second.

VII

The multiple realization argument is not the only objection to type materialism that is based on considerations having to do with multiple realization. In this section I will discuss two others. These objections are summarized by Block and Fodor in the following passages:

> First, the Lashleyan doctrine of neurological equipotentiality holds that any of a wide variety of psychological functions can be served by any of a wide variety of brain structures. While the generality of this doctrine may be disputed, it does seem clear that the central nervous system is highly labile and that a given type of psychological process is in fact often associated with a variety of distinct neurological structures. . . . Physicalism, as we have been construing it, requires that organisms are in type-identical psychological states if and only if they are in type-identical physical states. Hence, equipotentiality (if true) provides evidence against physicalism.

> [Second, psychological] similarities across species may often reflect convergent environmental selection rather than underlying physiological similarities. For example, we have no particular reason to suppose that the physiology of pain in man must have much in common with the physiology of pain in phylogenetically remote species. But if there are organisms whose psychology is homologous to our own but whose physiology is quite different, such organisms may provide counter-examples to the psychophysical correlations physicalism requires.[15]

15 See Ned Block and Jerry Fodor, "What Psychological States Are Not," *The Philosophical Review* 81 (1972), 159–81. The quoted passages occur on pages 160–61.

These objections will be called respectively the *equipotentiality argument* and the *appeal to other species*.

As it stands, the major premise of the equipotentiality argument is much too weak to bear its share of the weight of the conclusion. The major premise claims that a single qualitative kind may be associated with neurological states that differ in one or more fairly significant respects, and the conclusion claims that there are qualitative kinds that are not correlated with any one neurological kind. In order to obtain the conclusion, it is necessary to supplement the major premise with the thesis that state-tokens that differ in one or more significant respects cannot belong to a single neurological kind. That is to say, it is necessary to add the thesis that a neuroscientist is ex officio restricted to fine-grained principles of individuation for natural kinds. However, when one considers the variety of concepts that neuroscientists actually employ, and the variety of explanatory goals that they set themselves and occasionally reach, it becomes clear that they sometimes (though not always) use principles of individuation whose grain is extremely coarse. Neuroscience is concerned with understanding the structure and behavior of single cells and the interaction of small assemblies of cells, but it also recognizes the existence of large-scale mechanisms that involve scattered and gerrymandered collections of cells. It uses highly abstract structural and mathematical concepts in describing such mechanisms and in analyzing their behavior, and it also uses concepts from systems theory, communication theory, and computing. (Notice that concepts of these kinds are quite different from functional concepts.) A science that uses such concepts in picking out its kinds is fully capable of assigning states to a single natural kind even if the states differ in one or more significant respects.

In order to obtain the conclusion of the equipotentiality argument, it is not enough to appeal to a case in which a single qualitative characteristic is associated with two or more distinct neurophysiological state-types. One must go on to provide an exhaustive characterization of the distinct levels of description and explanation that belong to neuroscience, and show that no such level harbors a kind under which all of the states in question may be subsumed. I am not in a position to claim that it is impossible to accomplish these tasks, and I must therefore grant that there may be a version of the equipotentiality argument that is immune to the foregoing objection. I wish to claim only that no such version has yet appeared in the literature.

The appeal to other species suffers from two flaws, both of which have already been noted by Jaegwon Kim.[16] First, it suffers from the same flaw as the equipotentiality argument: As it stands, it fails to do justice to the fact that states can belong to a single natural kind even if they are quite different. Second, it presupposes that we can know that other organisms can have conscious experiences like ours even if they are quite remote from us, biologically speaking, and this presupposition is questionable. We have already found reasons to think that a rough, intuitive notion of biological similarity plays a role in the criteria that govern our third-person ascriptions, and we will find additional reasons in later chapters.

VIII

Although some behaviorists held that it is both possible and desirable to translate statements that purport to refer to sensations into statements that refer only to actual and potential behavior, others called for the elimination of such statements, claiming that our discourse about sensations is inextricably bound up with metaphysical beliefs about human beings that are best forgotten. Although it is no longer linked with behaviorism, which has fortunately worn out its welcome among philosophers and psychologists, the view that sensory concepts should be eliminated continues to attract adherents. Those who hold it today tend to call themselves *eliminative materialists*. They normally subscribe to the following propositions: (1) Our sensory concepts are implicitly defined by the laws of folk psychology, and accordingly they stand or fall with these laws; (2) folk psychology is an empirical theory; (3) because (2) is true, folk psychology is no less susceptible to revision and even elimination than the empirical theories that are devised by scientists; (4) the laws of folk psychology have flaws that are much too serious to be corrected by conceptual or logical surgery – they are incorrigibly flawed; (5) it is accordingly both possible and necessary to jettison the laws of folk psychology and their constituent concepts (including our sensory concepts); and (6) we should replace the jettisoned concepts with concepts borrowed from neuroscience.

In denying that our sensory concepts can be used to make statements that are literally true, eliminative materialists are in effect denying that it is appropriate to adopt a realist attitude toward sensations. Elimina-

16 See Jaegwon Kim, "Phenomenal Properties, Psychological Laws, and the Identity Theory," *The Monist* 56 (1972), 177–92.

tive materialism is, then, a form of anti-realism. It follows, of course, that if eliminative materialism is true, then type materialism must be false. Type materialism entails that sensations are every bit as real as trees and houses and stars.

What do eliminative materialists say in arguing for the extirpation of our sensory concepts? On what grounds are these concepts held to be defective? The argument that seems to have the greatest currency runs as follows:[17]

> **First premise.** The proposition that we are infallible with respect to our sensations is partially constitutive of our sensory concepts. (In other words: It is partially constitutive of our sensory concepts that it is possible to be certain of the existence and nature of one's sensations.)
>
> **Second premise.** Introspection is an instrument of limited scope and limited accuracy, and it is therefore false to say that we are infallible with respect to any of our internal states.
>
> **Conclusion.** Our sensory concepts are radically defective.

There is a certain tension between the premises of this argument. After all, one wonders, if introspection is as flawed as the second premise claims, how could we ever have adopted a conceptual scheme with the property cited in the first premise? Are we that stupid? However, the argument can be defended. As for the first premise, it seems that there are widely shared intuitions that attest to its truth. Thus, it has often been claimed in the history of philosophy that beliefs about sensations are certain or infallible. Authors of books and articles about sensations have often appealed to the infallibility of such beliefs in giving the defining features of their subject matter. What about the second premise? As I will argue in the next chapter, there is reason to believe that introspective judgments can go awry as a result of the influence of expectations upon belief-forming mechanisms. (Sometimes, I will argue, when one has been anticipating a sensation of type ϕ, and a sensation of another type occurs, one is led by one's expectations to believe, at least for a moment, that one's sensation is actually a sensation of type ϕ.) If my arguments in the next chapter are correct, it cannot be true that beliefs about sensations are infallible.

17 See, for example, section 3 of Daniel C. Dennett's "Quining Qualia," in A.J. Marcel and E. Bisiach (eds.), *Consciousness in Contemporary Science* (Oxford: Clarendon Press, 1988), pp. 42–77.

It is sometimes said that there is also a second reason for accepting the second premise – that it is possible to establish the fallibility of introspection by appealing to the fallibility of memory. Here, however, it is necessary to be careful. Let us say that a *transtemporal similarity judgment* is a judgment to the effect that one of one's current sensations stands in the relation of phenomenal similarity to one of one's past sensations. Now it is quite true that memory is fallible, and it is also true that we must rely on memory in making transtemporal similarity judgments. It follows that transtemporal similarity judgments are less than perfectly trustworthy. But this has no tendency to support the second premise. For the sort of infallibility that is in question there is infallibility with respect to one's current sensations. That is to say, the argument is concerned only with the epistemic status of purely introspective judgments. It is not concerned with the question of whether judgments based on introspection and memory can appropriately be regarded as infallible.

So what about it? Does the argument force us to adopt an anti-realist attitude toward sensations? No. Despite the fact that the first premise seems to be underwritten by intuitions that are widely shared, it is both possible and desirable to reject it. I think that the best way to show this is to develop a theory of introspective awareness that is obviously coherent and obviously well-motivated, and that implies (1) that beliefs about sensations are not certain or infallible, and (2) that such beliefs nevertheless have a very high degree of epistemic warrant. (Because of (2), a theory of this sort could be used to explain away the fact that beliefs about sensations seem to be infallible.) I will attempt to develop a theory with these features in the next chapter.

IX

Before bringing this defense of type materialism to a close, I will discuss an argument for eliminative materialism that is given in a recent paper by D.C. Dennett.[18] Dennett maintains that our sensory concepts give rise to questions that cannot be answered – even in principle. By using them, he claims, we generate puzzles and problems that are beyond the power of science to resolve. Seeing this as an undesirable feature of our conceptual scheme, he goes on to recommend that we replace our sensory concepts with new concepts that are better behaved.

18 Dennett, ibid., pp. 42–77.

Dennett's argument opens with a conversation between two coffee tasters who work for Maxwell House. One of the tasters, Mr. Chase, makes the following confession:

> I hate to admit it, but I'm not enjoying this work anymore. When I came to Maxwell House six years ago, I thought Maxwell House coffee was the best-tasting coffee in the world. I was proud to have a share in the responsibility for preserving that flavor over the years. And we've done our job well; the coffee tastes just the same today as it tasted when I arrived. But, you know, I no longer like it! My tastes have changed. I've become a more sophisticated coffee drinker. I no longer like *that taste* at all.[19]

The second taster, Mr. Sanborn, gives this response:

> When I arrived here, shortly before you did, I, like you, thought Maxwell House coffee was tops in flavor. And now I, like you, really don't care for the coffee we're making. But *my* tastes haven't changed; my . . . *tasters* have changed. That is, I think something has gone wrong with my taste buds or some other part of my taste-analyzing perceptual machinery. Maxwell House coffee doesn't taste to me the way it used to taste; if only it did, I'd still love it, for I still think *that taste* is the best taste in coffee. Now I'm not saying we haven't done our job well. You other tasters all agree that the taste is the same, and I must admit that on a day-to-day basis I can detect no change either. So it must be my problem alone. I guess I'm no longer cut out for this work.[20]

Chase and Sanborn provide us with interpretations of the data that they are given by introspection and memory. We are initially inclined, perhaps, to accept their interpretations as being substantially correct. However, as Dennett points out, other interpretations are possible. Take Chase. One interpretation is the interpretation that he favors – namely, that his aesthetic standards have changed. But there is a second interpretation. It is possible that Chase has undergone a transformation like the one that Sanborn claims that *he* has undergone, but that Chase's memories have changed in such a way as to make it seem that his taste qualia are still correlated with external stimuli in the way that they have always been. (We can suppose that the change in Chase's taste qualia has been sufficiently gradual to escape his notice.) And there is a third interpretation. It is possible that there have been changes in all

19 Dennett, ibid., p. 52.
20 Dennett, ibid., p. 52.

three of the relevant variables. Thus, it may be that Chase's aesthetic standards have changed, but not as much as he thinks, and that the difference between this change in his aesthetic standards and the perceived change in his enjoyment of Maxwell House coffee is to be attributed to a combination of a change in qualia (that is, a change of the sort that Sanborn describes, but of lesser degree) and a memory change.

We can, following Dennett, reformulate these hypotheses as follows:

> (a) As Chase himself believes, his dispositions to produce qualitative states have remained intact, but his dispositions to react to already-produced qualitative states have undergone a substantial transformation. (His dispositions to react include dispositions to make aesthetic judgments about qualitative states and memory-based dispositions to make comparative judgments concerning current qualitative states and qualitative states of the past.)

> (b) Chase's reactive dispositions have remained constant, but his dispositions to generate qualia have changed.

> (c) Chase's generative dispositions have changed, but only slightly, and his reactive dispositions have undergone slight changes as well.

There are, of course, three similar hypotheses about Sanborn.

Once Dennett has set out the alternative hypothesis, he goes on to make three observations.

The first is that Chase is unable to determine which of the hypotheses is correct on the basis of introspection and memory alone. (The same applies to Sanborn.) Chase appears to be confident that (a) is true; but if he is going only on how things seem from the inside, he has no right to feel such confidence. For (b) and (c) are fully compatible with all of the data that are provided by introspection and memory. In order to reach a well-grounded decision, Chase must obtain information from some other source.

Generalizing, we can put the point as follows: There are questions about one's inner world that cannot be settled by the information that is available to one qua occupant of that world.

Dennett's second point is that Chase may be able to improve his epistemic position vis-à-vis the competing hypotheses by obtaining information of the sort that is available to external observers. Specifically, Chase may be able to find behavioral or neurological evidence that tends to confirm one of the two extreme hypotheses (namely, (a) and (b)) at the expense of the other.

> Thus if Chase is unable to reidentify coffees, teas, and wines in blind tastings in which only minutes intervene between first and second sips, his claim to *know* that Maxwell House tastes just the same to him now as it did six years ago will be seriously undercut. Alternatively, if he does excellently in blind tastings, and exhibits considerable knowledge about the canons of coffee style (if such there be), his claim to have become a more sophisticated taster will be supported. . . . And as Shoemaker . . . and others have noted, physiological measures, suitably interpreted in some larger theoretical framework, could also weight the scales in favor of one extreme or the other.[21]

Here, then, are several ways in which information about the external world can help one to resolve questions about the internal world. As Dennett notes, the possibility that it is sometimes necessary to obtain such information has been pretty much ignored within the Cartesian tradition.

Dennett's third point is that behavioral and neurological information will inevitably leave a certain amount of slack. Such information may be able to rule out (a) or (b), he says, but it cannot provide grounds for choosing between the surviving member of this pair and a suitably formulated version of (c). He writes:

> But let us not overestimate the resolving power of such empirical testing. The space between the two poles represented by possibility (a) and possibility (b) would be occupied by phenomena that were the product, somehow, of two factors in varying proportion: roughly, dispositions to generate or produce qualia and dispositions to react to the qualia once they are produced. (That is how our intuitive picture of qualia would envisage it.) Qualia are supposed to affect our action or behavior only via the intermediary of our judgments about them, so any behavioral test, such as a discrimination or memory test, since it takes acts based on judgments as its primary data, can give us direct evidence only about the *resultant* of our two factors. In extreme cases we can have indirect evidence to suggest that one factor has varied a great deal, the other factor hardly at all, and we can test the hypothesis further by checking the relative sensitivity of the subject to variations in the conditions that presumably alter the two component factors. But such indirect testing

---

21 Dennett, ibid., pp. 55–56.

cannot be expected to resolve the issue when the effects are relatively small – when, for instance, our rival hypotheses are Chase's preferred hypothesis (a) and the minor variant to the effect that his qualia have shifted *a little* and his standards *less than he thinks.*[22]

Dennett is here concerned primarily with behavioral data, but he thinks that the same points apply, mutatis mutandis, to information about neural states. Presumably he would try to justify this view in something like the following way: Our evidence for correlations between neural states and qualitative states is always indirect. Thus, consider an experimental setup that is designed to give us information about correlations of the sort in question. A subject in an experiment of this kind must take note of his or her qualitative states in order to provide evidence of their occurrence. This means that the evidence that is obtained will be, in the first instance, evidence concerning correlations between neural states and *judgments about* qualitative states. But now, judgments about qualitative states are always produced jointly by two factors, generative dispositions and reactive dispositions. Accordingly, we would have to factor out the contributions made by reactive dispositions in order to reach any conclusions about relationships between neural states and qualitative states. And how would we do that? To succeed, we would need to have some sort of independent access to qualitative states. But it is precisely because there is no such access that we are now trying to get a fix on qualitative states by exploiting neurosensory correlations.

What conclusions should we draw from Dennett's argument? As I see it, he makes a strong case for his first point, the claim that there are questions about the phenomenal world that cannot be settled on the basis of introspection and memory alone. I also feel that we should accept his second point: We should agree that it is sometimes possible to improve one's epistemic situation vis-à-vis hypotheses about the internal world by obtaining behavioral and neurological data.

What about Dennett's third point? Has he established that there are questions about qualitative states that cannot be settled by appealing either to internal evidence or to external evidence? Is it true that there are questions about qualitative states that cannot be settled at all – even in principle? Here, I feel, it would be a mistake to acquiesce in Dennett's reasoning. I have three objections.

22 Dennett, ibid., pp. 22–23.

In the first place, insofar as Dennett's case depends on the claim that it is impossible to find evidence that enables us to choose between hypotheses about qualia that are very close to one another in content, I feel that he has no case at all. Evidence always leaves a certain amount of slack in science. This is why we hear so much about simplicity and other nonevidential determinants of theory choice. Accordingly, if an inability to choose between hypotheses that are very close in content was a good reason for jettisoning our sensory concepts, we would be obliged to dispense with concepts that stand for physical properties and relations as well. But this is wild! There may be considerations that will one day force us to renounce the latter concepts, but our inability to choose between close hypotheses is not among them.

Second, it is a mistake to claim that "qualia are supposed to affect our action or behavior only via the intermediary of our judgments about them," and by the same token, it is a mistake to suppose that our access to qualitative states is always mediated by judgments. The extent to which relationships between qualitative states and behavior are mediated by judgments depends upon what one means by "judgment." However, on any reasonable construal of the term, it is clear that in many cases no such mediation occurs. In many cases the path leading from a sensation to behavior is direct.

Third, although it is true that a variety of reactive dispositions play important roles in the production of judgments about qualitative states, and true, therefore, that evidence concerning neurosensory correlations requires a certain amount of interpretation, it is also true that we are to a large extent able to factor out the contributions of the various reactive dispositions. This is because it is not the case that every sort of reactive disposition plays a role in the production of every judgment. As a result of this fact, where D is a typical reactive disposition, it is possible to distinguish between neural states that are correlated with D-influenced judgments and neural states that are correlated with judgments that are independent of D.

But is it really true that the influence of reactive dispositions is limited in this way? Of course! For example, take the family of reactive dispositions with which Dennett is primarily concerned – the dispositions that are based on memory. There is no reason to think that memory always plays an active role in the production of judgments about qualitative states. Thus, there is no reason to think that it plays an active role in the production of simple classificatory judgments that are concerned with currently existing sensations, nor in the production of similarity judgments about coexisting sensations. Why should it? After all, the content of such judgments has nothing to do with the past. (To be sure, judgments about our current sensations commit us to judgments that compare current sensations with past sensations; but this is quite different than making a claim about the past.)[23]

23 It may be true that memory always plays a role in the production of qualitative states themselves (as opposed to playing a role in the production of judgments about qualitative states), but any contribution of this sort would be irrelevant to the questions that are before us now. This is because any such contribution would be on the generative side of the generative/reactive boundary. Our concern here is whether it is possible to get at the outputs of the generative dispositions by factoring out the effects of the reactive dispositions.

PART THREE

Introspection

5

Introspective awareness of sensations

In this chapter I will distinguish between several forms of introspective awareness of sensations and give an account of their most basic properties. My goal is to formulate a theory of introspection that can be integrated with the reductionist view of sensations that I have defended in earlier chapters.

I will also develop a skeletal theory of the epistemological status of introspective beliefs about sensations. It is often claimed in philosophy that all such beliefs are infallible, and that the scope of introspection is sufficiently comprehensive that we can be said to be omniscient with respect to the realm of sensations. I will argue that these claims are much too strong, but I will also maintain that they contain an element of truth. I will conclude with a brief discussion of the question of what we mean when we describe an introspective belief as justified.

I

Frequently, when we say that a subject is introspectively aware of a sensation of type ϕ, we are making a claim that has the following truth conditions: (1) S has a sensation of type ϕ; (2) S believes that he or she has a sensation of type ϕ; and (3) the belief cited in (2) is both caused and confirmed by the sensation cited in (1). When a claim of this sort is true, S has what I call *basic awareness* of one of his or her sensations.

Basic awareness is a form of consciousness. Thus, according to the definition, to be in a state of basic awareness is to stand in a certain epistemic relation to a sensation. It is to have knowledge of the existence of a sensation on the basis of one's current experience. But

This chapter owes much to Sydney Shoemaker. I have been helped considerably both by conversations with him and by the lectures he gave in the summer of 1985 in his N.E.H. Summer Seminar on Self-Consciousness and Self-Reference. I have also received valuable advice from Carolyn Black, Anthony Brueckner, Willem de Vries, Ivan Fox, William G. Lycan, David Roach, David A. Schroeder, Thomas Senor, and David H. Westendorf. Large portions of sections I–IV are excerpted from my "Introspective Awareness of Sensations," *Topoi* 6 (1987), 9–22.

117

there is a sense of "conscious" in which it expresses this very epistemic relation. In general, when someone has knowledge of the existence of something by virtue of his or her current experience, it is appropriate to say that he or she is *conscious of* that thing. At the present moment, for example, it is appropriate to say that I am conscious of the pen in my hand.

Basic awareness differs from perceptual awareness in a respect that is of great importance. Let us say that a *state of awareness* is a belief together with any sense experiences that both occur at the same time as the belief and serve as evidence that it is true. In the case of perception, a state of awareness is directed on an object that is altogether external to the state itself. The object of awareness cannot be said to be a constituent of the state of awareness. But we find a quite different situation when we consider basic awareness. In this case, the entity that serves as the object of awareness is identical with the sensory component of the state of awareness. The object of awareness is included in the state of awareness.

II

There is no clause in the definition of basic awareness that indicates that it calls for an action of any kind: Basic awareness is an essentially passive phenomenon. But our ordinary discourse testifies to the existence of a form of introspective awareness that is essentially active in nature. Thus, we are disposed to describe ourselves and others as "attending to an itch," "concentrating on a toothache," "focusing on a burning sensation," and "scrutinizing a taste." Attending counts intuitively as an action, and so do concentrating, focusing, and scrutinizing.

It is, I believe, possible to distinguish between three forms of active introspection. I call them *inner vision, volume adjustment*, and *activation*.

Inner vision occurs when one decides to attend to a sensation that is already in existence but that has not yet been subjected to scrutiny. The sensation itself is not altered in any way by one's coming to attend to it. Rather there is a change in one's cognitive attitude toward the sensation: One takes an interest in its components and their properties, and one undertakes to distinguish between the components and to assign them to the appropriate categories. The upshot is a new set of introspective beliefs – a new set of states of basic awareness.

It is quite clear, I think, that there is such a thing as a sensation of which one is not aware (an unconscious sensation, if you like), and, by the same token, that there is such a thing as coming to be aware of a sensation that was in existence prior to one's state of awareness.[1] Here is an example: As I pace back and forth in my room I find that I frequently pause in front of the window. Asking myself why, it suddenly dawns on me that I am quite cold, and that my pauses have been due to the succoring warmth of the sun's rays. A second example: I find myself scratching one of my legs and come to realize that I am doing so for a reason – the leg is itching.[2]

What happens in cases of inner vision? How should we conceptualize the form of attention that is found in such cases? These questions are answered – albeit in a very rough and preliminary way – by a theory I call the *inner eye hypothesis*.

The inner eye hypothesis maintains that there is a level of representation that mediates between sensations and beliefs about sensations. The representations at this level are said to be states of an internal scanning device, and this scanning device is said to stand in much the same relationship to sensations as the physical eye does to extramental objects and events. One attends to an extramental entity by arranging for one's physical eye to be in the right position to pick up information about the entity. It is much the same, according to the inner eye hypothesis, in the case of introspection: One attends to a sensation by adjusting one's internal scanning device in such a way that it becomes attuned to information about the sensation. Further, extramental entities can exist without standing in any informational relations to the physical eye, and their internal qualities are never affected by their coming to stand in such relations. The inner eye hypothesis claims that the same things are true, mutatis mutandis, of sensations and one's internal scanning device. It asserts that sensations can exist without being scanned, and also that the internal qualities of sensations do not change when one scans them.

The inner eye hypothesis does not identify the state of being aware of a sensation with a state of one's scanner. The hypothesis claims that being aware of a sensation is a matter of having a belief. (Specifically, it claims that awareness of a sensation is a matter of having a belief that is at once caused and confirmed by the sensation itself.) The scanner is a device for picking up and sorting information, and as such it plays a

---

1 Other examples of "unconscious" sensations are given in the antepenultimate paragraph of section IV.
2 Armstrong has called attention to a different but closely related phenomenon. See David M. Armstrong, *The Nature of Mind* (Ithaca: Cornell University Press, 1981), 59.

role in producing beliefs. But one cannot be said to have an introspective belief simply by virtue of the fact that one's scanner is in a certain state.

Volume adjustment is like inner vision in that it involves taking an interest in a sensation that is already in existence. It is different, however, in that one adjusts the volume of a sensation by changing it in certain ways. One wants to bring the sensation into greater prominence in the phenomenal field, and this desire leads one to take steps to heighten the intensity of the sensation or to increase its degree of internal articulation. As in the case of inner vision, the final stage of volume adjustment is the production of a set of new states of basic awareness. It is by virtue of these states that volume adjustment can be said to involve awareness of sensations. (The name "volume adjustment" derives from the similarity between changing the intensity of a sensation and changing the volume of the sounds emanating from a radio.[3])

Volume adjustment is a familiar phenomenon. Suppose, for example, that you are a dinner guest, and that because you are seated next to a gifted raconteur, you have neglected to attend to the taste of your coq au vin. Realizing suddenly that it is time to compliment your host, you withdraw from the conversation and focus for a moment on your gustatory sensations. This shift in your attention will very likely add considerably to the intensity of the sensations, and it may also cause them to acquire a number of facets or aspects that they had previously lacked. Changes of these two kinds count as changes in prominence.

I have said that an increase in prominence involves changes along one or both of two distinguishable dimensions – intensity and degree of internal articulation. But what is intensity? It seems to mean different things in different cases. Attention can increase the phenomenal volume of an auditory sensation, the vividness of a gustatory sensation, the severity of a pain, the importunity of an itch, and the strength of a feeling of pressure. I am strongly inclined to view these changes as similar, and it seems natural to use "intensity" as a label for the respect of comparison in terms of which their similarity is to be understood. However, in view of the obvious differences between such dimensions

---

3 The idea of drawing an analogy between attending to sensations and adjusting the volume of a radio is due to D.C. Dennett. See "Why You Can't Make a Computer that Feels Pain" in Dennett's *Brainstorms* (Cambridge, MA: MIT Press, 1978), 190–229. See especially p. 202.

as phenomenal volume and severity of pain, the claim that they are similar is badly in need of clarification and defense. Unfortunately, I am not in a position to give an account of this matter here.

What happens when a sensation undergoes an increase in internal articulation?[4] Among other things, a change of this sort may involve the emergence of more minute details, a reduction in the fuzziness of details that are already at hand, a strengthening of the ties between constituents that are organized into *gestalten* (with an accompanying heightening of the salience of these *gestalten*), and the appearance of new *gestalt* phenomena as a result of the aforementioned changes. However, these are only examples. I am unable to give a full analysis of internal articulation.

It is no doubt true that when one engages in volume adjustment one sometimes performs the same actions as when one engages in inner vision. In addition to the activities associated with increasing the intensity and the internal articulation of a sensation, it may be necessary to tune or change the orientation of one's internal scanner to enable it to pick up the new information that comes into existence as the sensation becomes more prominent. (It may also be true that inner vision typically involves some of the activities that are associated with volume adjustment. It may be the case that there are two sets of activities, or two sets of mechanisms, that are involved in inner vision and volume adjustment, and that the difference between these two forms of active introspection is simply a matter of degree to which each depends on the activities or mechanisms in one of the two sets rather than the other.)

This brings us to activation. It often happens that one has a description of a type of sensation in mind and one undertakes to determine whether it is currently possible to bring a sensation answering to that description to the surface of consciousness. Activation occurs if one succeeds in actualizing or activating a sensation of the right sort. Thus, for example, having lost touch with the aftertaste of one's most recent cup of coffee as a result of being temporarily preoccupied with other matters, one might suddenly recall the aftertaste and undertake to determine whether it is possible to experience it anew. After turning one's attention to the area of phenomenal space in which taste sensations are encountered, one might experience the gradual rebirth of the aftertaste. Here is another example: "If you will attend fixedly for a

4 I owe the term "internal articulation" to Fox.

few moments to any point on the external skin, you will find coming into consciousness a number of itching, tingling, or prickling sensations which you had not previously noticed, and would in all probability not have observed were it not for the increased attention to that part of the body."[5]

What happens when one attempts to summon a sensation answering to some description into one's phenomenal field? I am not in a position to specify the underlying mechanisms, but I think it is not difficult to see what form the answer must take. It is natural to suppose that each sensation derives ultimately from a packet of information in an unconscious portion of one's mind – a packet that has the potential to become a sensation with a particular set of phenomenal characteristics, but that must be subjected to further processing before it can achieve its potential. If this is right, the task of summoning a sensation of a certain kind into existence must have the following two steps. First, one attempts to determine whether there is an unconscious packet of information that is of the right kind to produce a sensation answering to the description one has in mind. Second, in the event that a packet of the right kind is available, one adjusts the controls that activate the appropriate information-processing mechanisms, and the packet is converted into a sensation. In short, one summons a sensation of a certain kind into existence by actualizing the potential of a packet of information of the right sort. (The activities involved in this process are of course largely unconscious.)

In its present guise the account of active introspection that I have been developing is less a theory than a set of rather sketchy metaphors. To proceed beyond the metaphorical level, it would be necessary to address a number of extremely difficult questions. I have said that I am not in a position to answer these questions. It should be mentioned, however, that it is possible to find a certain amount of relevant information elsewhere in the literature.[6,7]

5 See W.B. Pillsbury, *Attention* (New York: Macmillan, 1908), 6. I take it that the kind of case Pillsbury is describing here is different from the kind of case in which one finds oneself scratching a leg, and then notices that the leg is itching. In the former case, one notices a phenomenal change; one experiences the birth of an itch. In the latter case, one does not. At most there is an increase in prominence.

6 Not surprisingly, there are some interesting discussions of the changes in the phenomenal field that accompany attention in the writings of such introspectionist psychologists as James, Wundt, Titchener, and Pillsbury. (Some of these discussions provide fairly

III

Although philosophers have written at length about the phenomenon I have called inner vision, and have often endorsed versions of the inner eye hypothesis, they have had very little to say about the phenomena I have called volume adjustment and activation. There has been little recognition of the fact that a sensation may be transformed by the act of coming to attend to it, and even less of the fact that a sensation may be brought into existence by attention. Instead of facing these facts and attempting to explain them, philosophers have often waged an imperialist struggle on behalf of inner vision and the inner eye hypothesis. They have maintained, either explicitly or implicitly, that inner vision is the only important form of active introspection, and they have attempted to deny or to reinterpret the data that are incompatible with

---

strong support for my contention that the prominence of sensations can be analyzed in terms of intensity and degree of internal articulation.) See, for example, the following works: William James, *The Principles of Psychology*, Vol. I (New York: Dover Publications, 1950), 402–58; Wilhelm Wundt, *Outlines of Psychology*, 3rd English edition (Leipzig: Alfred Kroner, 1907), 228–51; Edward B. Titchener, *A Text-Book of Psychology*, revised edition (New York: Macmillan, 1909), 53–54 and 265–83; and W.B. Pillsbury, op. cit. 2–10. For a survey of the literature about one of the key concepts in nineteenth-century discussions of attention, see I.M. Bentley, "The Psychological Meaning of Clearness," *Mind* XIII (1904): 242–53.

7 Given that contemporary psychologists are often reluctant to become deeply involved in issues concerning qualitatively individuated states, it is natural to assume that it will be some time before modern psychology provides any information about the information-processing mechanisms that underlie active introspection. However, this assumption is not quite true. Cognitive psychologists are concerned to explain what is involved in attending to extramental objects and events, and some of their findings have an indirect bearing on questions about attending to sensations. According to cognitive psychology, attending to an extramental entity should be seen as a matter of committing a sense receptor and one or more information-processing mechanisms to the task of obtaining a detailed and trustworthy representation of the entity. (See, for example, the following papers: Donald E. Broadbent, "Task Combination and Selective Intake of Information," *Acta Psychologica* 50 (1982): 253–90; Daniel Kahneman and Anne Triesman, "Changing Views of Attention and Automaticity," in Raja Parasuraman and D.R. Davies (eds.), *Varieties of Attention* (New York: Academic Press, 1984), 29–61; William A. Johnston and Veronica J. Dark, "Selective Attention," *Annual Review of Psychology* 37 (1986): 43–75.) Because the task of obtaining a detailed and trustworthy representation of an extramental entity consists partly in obtaining a prominent sensation that represents the entity, and because changes in prominence are partially constitutive of attending to sensations, it is appropriate to say that theories about the information-processing mechanisms that underlie attending to extramental objects and events are implicitly germane to certain aspects of active introspection.

123

this view. Correlatively, they have urged that the inner eye hypothesis gives a more or less complete picture of the processes and mechanisms that are involved in active introspection.[8]

Why have philosophers been attracted by this form of imperialism? It can seem that inner vision is the only form of active introspection that is fully compatible with our intuitions about what happens when we introspect. When I bring an already familiar sensation into greater prominence I never consciously think of myself as changing its intrinsic qualities, and when I undertake to summon up a new sensation I do not normally think of myself as undertaking to bring a sensation into existence. Rather I think of myself as "taking a closer look" at a sensation, or as "looking for" a sensation of a particular kind.

It seems, then, that we normally conceptualize the process of attending to sensations in terms of a perceptual model. However, although this point may enable us to understand the appeal of imperialism, it has no tendency whatsoever to show that imperialism is sound. Thus, it by no means follows that it is in any deep sense correct to conceptualize attending to sensations in terms of a perceptual model, or even that we believe it to be deeply correct to do so. The fact is that we find it natural to describe a number of different phenomena in terms of perceptual models. We do not find it natural to use such models because we sense that there are deep underlying similarities between perception and the phenomena we are describing. There are similarities, of course, but they tend to be rather superficial. We notice them only because sense perception is never very far from our thoughts.

Think of a laboratory technician who is trying to determine the composition of a sample by chemical analysis. The technician may find it perfectly natural to say that he or she is "taking a closer look" at the sample. In saying this, however, the technician does not mean to assert that he or she is doing something that is fundamentally akin to what we do when we subject an object to closer visual scrutiny. When one subjects an object to closer visual scrutiny, one simply changes the

8 There is a danger here for those with a penchant for championing the underdog: In one's eagerness to come to the defense of volume adjustment and activation, one may fail to do justice to inner vision. I succumbed to this danger in a paper that was in effect an early draft of this chapter. Thus, in "Introspective Awareness of Sensation" (*Topoi* 6 (1987), 9–22) I ignored the data that attest to the existence of inner vision, and I argued that the inner eye hypothesis fails to describe *any* of the mechanisms or processes that are involved in active introspection. A chapter in Lycan's *Consciousness* has convinced me that this was a mistake. (See W.G. Lycan, *Consciousness* (Cambridge, MA: MIT Press, 1987), Chapter 6.)

relation between the object and one's eyes. But a technician who is analyzing a sample may well be changing many of its intrinsic qualities.

I see no reason to prefer imperialism to the view that the phenomenal field is often profoundly changed by the process of coming to attend to a sensation. But more: It seems to me that there is a strong reason to accept this second view. I will now try to show that there are data that imperialism is incapable of accommodating.

Attending to a sensation often involves one or more introspectible changes in the internal qualities of sensations. Thus, consider a case in which someone decides to focus on a sensation that has heretofore been at the margin of consciousness. If the sensation is an itch, attending to it may make it more importunate; if it is a pain, attending to it may make it more severe; if it is an auditory sensation, attending to it may increase its phenomenal volume; if it is a visual sensation, attending to it may increase its vividness; and so on.

Now the inner eye hypothesis describes active introspection as a process that involves the following stages: First, one adjusts the orientation of one's internal scanning device; second, the device picks up new information about a sensation somewhere in one's phenomenal field; third, the device enters an internal state that counts as a representation of the sensation; and fourth, this representation causes one to form one or more beliefs about the sensation. (In a case in which one is attending more closely to an already familiar sensation the representation is a new and improved version of a prior representation, and in a case in which one is attending to a new sensation the representation differs in character and content from all of its immediate predecessors.) According to the imperialist, it is possible to give a complete account of active introspection without postulating any events beyond the events associated with these four stages. In particular, it is possible to give a complete account without claiming that active introspection brings about changes in the internal qualities of sensations.

As this account shows, the imperialist claims that attending to a sensation is ultimately a matter of forming a representation of the sensation. How then can imperialism do justice to the fact that attending to a sensation normally involves introspectible changes? It can do so only by claiming that the process of forming a representation of a sensation is itself an introspectible change. It follows that imperialism is committed to *two* levels of introspectible states. One level consists of sensations, and the other consists of the states of one's internal scanning device that count as representations of sensations.

We are now in a position to see that imperialism is badly flawed. First, it runs afoul of the principle of simplicity that counsels us to eschew duplications of kinds of entities unless they are forced on us by data or by systematic considerations. (It is clear that there is nothing that forces us to claim the existence of two separate levels of introspectible states.) Second, imperialism misdescribes the "location" of the introspectible changes that occur when one engages in active introspection. The introspectible changes that occur when one attends to a sensation are changes in the qualitative nature of the sensation to which one is attending. (Thus, for example, as we noticed earlier, attending to an itch normally brings about an increase in importunity. It is clear that a change of this sort is a change in the qualitative nature of the sensation that is the object of one's attention.) It follows immediately that imperialism is mistaken, for it implies that the introspectible changes associated with active introspection do not involve sensations but rather the states of one's inner scanning device by which sensations are represented.

I have been arguing that there are data that the imperialist cannot explain. The argument has been based on cases that suggest that there is such a thing as volume adjustment – that is, on cases in which a qualitative change occurs when one directs one's attention on a sensation that has previously been at the margin of consciousness. But it is also possible to cause problems for imperialism by appealing to the data that suggest that there is such a thing as activation. Consider what it is like to attend to a sensation that has not previously been an object of awareness. Sometimes when one turns one's attention to a new region of phenomenal space, one has the sense that one is making the acquaintance of a sensation that has been in existence for some time. But on other occasions one experiences the gradual dawning of a new sensation; one is aware of the eruption of a new sensation into one's phenomenal field. Cases of this second sort are flatly incompatible with the imperialist's contention that inner vision is the only form of active introspection.

IV

Since Descartes, philosophical discussions of introspective beliefs about sensations have tended to focus on two principles about the epistemological status of such beliefs. These principles may be expressed as follows:

It is logically necessary that if p is a proposition to the effect that S currently has a sensation with a certain phenomenal quality, and S believes that p, then it is true that p.

It is logically necessary that if p is a proposition to the effect that S currently has a sensation with a certain phenomenal quality, and it is true that p, then S believes that p.

The first principle, which I call the *infallibility thesis*, claims that our beliefs about the phenomenal qualities of our sensations are necessarily free from error. The other principle asserts that our knowledge of the phenomenal qualities of our sensations is necessarily complete. Following Armstrong, I call this second principle the *self-intimation thesis*.[9]

In order to appreciate the appeal of these principles it is helpful to contemplate one of the main differences between perceptual beliefs about extramental phenomena and introspective beliefs about sensations. In dealing with extramental phenomena we frequently have occasion to contrast appearance with reality. The relationship between extramental phenomena and our beliefs about them involves qualitatively individuated representations (that is, sensations) that count as appearances, and these appearances can be misleading in a number of ways. However, it is at once a teaching of common sense and a consequence of the theory of introspection presented in the previous sections that there is no appearance/reality distinction in the case of sensations. There is no set of appearances that mediate between sensations and our beliefs about them. In the case of sensations the appearance *is* the reality. This fact can seem to exclude erroneous judgments about sensations and also ignorance of their phenomenal qualities. How could we form false beliefs about sensations if there are no misleading appearances to betray us? And how could we fail to be aware of our sensations if there is no distinction between the sensations that exist and the sensations that put in an appearance?

I acknowledge the force of this argument. In my judgment, it shows that the infallibility thesis and the self-intimation thesis both contain important elements of truth. Nevertheless, I think it is necessary to

9 See D.M. Armstrong, *A Materialist Theory of the Mind* (London: Routledge and Kegan Paul, 1968), 101. (Armstrong tells us that he borrowed the term from Ryle.)

Despite the fact that Armstrong's theory about the nature of introspection appears to be quite different than the theory I develop in sections I–III (he favors a version of imperialism), his views about the epistemological status of introspective beliefs are quite similar to the views that are expressed in section IV. (I have found it extremely helpful to consult his writings on introspection in developing my own position.)

reject these principles. I will give grounds for rejecting them in the following paragraphs, and I will then attempt to state new principles that lack their flaws but that also capture the parts of their content that are true.

In order to assess the infallibility thesis adequately, it is necessary to distinguish between two kinds of errors that we are prone to make. First, as we have just noticed, errors can occur when beliefs are based on appearances that fail to do justice to the entities to which the beliefs refer. When we are misled in this way by imperfect information, we make errors that may be called *errors of ignorance*. Second, errors can arise when we have adequate information about the entities with which we are concerned but we fail to take this information fully into account in forming beliefs about the entities. Errors of this sort, which may be called *errors of judgment*, are usually due either to some form of inattention or to the influence of expectation upon judgment. They tend to occur when we are hasty in forming beliefs, when we are suffering from information overload, when we are preoccupied, and when we are being lazy. They also tend to occur in situations in which anticipation causes us to lower the thresholds of application that are associated with some of our concepts.

Although we are perforce innocent of committing errors of ignorance in forming beliefs about our own sensations, we do run the risk of misconstruing our sensations by committing errors of judgment. Take the phenomenal quality *being a tactual sensation that consists of twelve pinprick sensations*. One might misclassify an instance of this quality as a sensation consisting of eleven pinprick sensations if one were forced to reach a conclusion about its complexity in a hurry, and one might also do so if one were concerned with other matters at the time. Further, one might misclassify an instance if one had been given reason in advance to expect that one's next tactual sensation would have twelve components. This example involves phenomenal qualities that are fairly complex – that is, qualities that cannot be apprehended without doing more information processing than the bare minimum. But it is also possible to commit errors of judgment in forming beliefs about *simple* qualities of sensations, such as the quality *being a pain*. My favorite example is a case that was presented by Rogers Albritton a number of years ago in a seminar. This case involves a college student who is being initiated into a fraternity. He is shown a razor, and is then blindfolded and told that the razor will be drawn across his throat. When he feels a sensation he cries out: He believes for a split second that he is in pain.

However, after contemplating the sensation for a moment, he comes to feel that it is actually an experience of some other kind. It is, he decides, a sensation of cold. And this belief is confirmed when, a bit later, the blindfold is removed and he is shown that his throat is in contact with an icicle rather than a razor.

In addition to more or less anecdotal arguments of this sort, which provide grounds for thinking that it is both logically and nomologically possible for there to be erroneous beliefs about sensations, there are grounds for thinking that we often form such beliefs (or at least, that we are disposed to form them) in the actual world. Thus, there is evidence – indirect, but nonetheless strong – that we are prone to misclassify sensations that are markedly similar. It is well established that subjects in experiments frequently confuse similar colors, similar tones, similar tastes, and so on.[10] These findings do not count directly in favor of the claim that we are prone to confuse similar sensations, for the subjects in question are typically asked to concern themselves with external stimuli. However, their judgments about stimuli may be taken as evidence concerning their dispositions to make judgments about sensations. They would hardly be capable of confusing two stimuli if they were disposed to make fully accurate judgments about the sensations to which the stimuli correspond.

It appears, then, that the infallibility thesis is wrong. What about the self-intimation thesis? There are a number of reasons for thinking that it is no more worthy of our assent than the infallibility thesis. I will cite three of them.

First, errors of judgment count no less heavily against the self-intimation thesis than against the infallibility thesis. When one makes an error of judgment one forms a false belief. But more: One also fails to form a true belief. Failures of this sort are counterexamples to the self-intimation thesis. Second, inattention often keeps us from forming beliefs about a number of the details of our visual sensations. Often, when we consider our beliefs about a recent visual sensation, we find that we have firm beliefs about the components to which we have

10 Psychophysicists have long found it necessary to allow for a variety of errors in establishing absolute thresholds and difference thresholds. Here is a typical observation: "One sticky problem, though, for the concept of the threshold is that of judgement errors. All of the psychophysical methods that have been discussed [in this text] have some procedure for balancing out 'errors' in judgement that may interfere with the observer's ability to report accurately his sensory experiences." See Ronald H. Forgus and Lawrence E. Melamed, *Perception*, 2nd edition (New York: McGraw-Hill, 1976), 38.

attended but only the vaguest idea as to identities of the other components. Third, it seems that human beings are sometimes unable to apprehend their sensations because they lack the conceptual resources to do so. Consider, for example, a young baby who encounters a gustatory sensation that has a number of characteristics with which it is not yet fully familiar. Not many of us would want to maintain that all of the aspects of this sensation can be known with certainty. For knowledge requires the possession of concepts, and by hypothesis the baby is too unsophisticated to have concepts of the phenomenal qualities that represent certain aspects of its current sensation. For the same reason, few of us would want to maintain that the baby is able to form beliefs that do full justice to the distinctive natures of all of the aspects. (If one were to insist that the baby has a fund of concepts that is adequate to represent all of the aspects, one would have to defend either the view that all of our concepts of phenomenal qualities are a priori, or the view that a baby can devise or refine a number of new concepts at exactly the same time as it is deploying the concepts in forming beliefs. Neither of these views has much intuitive appeal.)

The infallibility thesis and the self-intimation thesis are much too strong, but it would be a mistake to abandon them altogether. The appearance/reality argument that we considered at the beginning of this section shows that they are not completely lacking in merit. I suggest that they should be replaced with two principles that I call respectively the *direct awareness thesis* and the *manifest nature thesis*:

> It is nomologically necessary that if x believes that y has a certain phenomenal quality, where y is one of x's current sensations, and x's belief is based on y, then x has not been misled by appearances.

> It is nomologically necessary that if (1) p is a proposition to the effect that y has a certain phenomenal quality, where y is one of x's current sensations, (2) it is true that p, (3) x believes either p or the denial of p, (4) this belief is based on y, (5) x has not committed an error of judgment, and (6) x has not been misled by faulty memories of past sensations, then x believes that p.

These principles may require some minor qualifications. However, as far as I have been able to determine, they are refreshingly free from major flaws. (Why the shift to nomological necessity? The answer is that the theses hold by virtue of certain facts about the relationships between human cognitive mechanisms. Facts of this sort are logically contingent.)

V

We will now consider a feature of the foregoing account of introspection that may have been bothering the reader for some time. The account is based largely on my description of basic awareness, and that description presupposes that beliefs about sensations can meaningfully be said to be confirmed or justified by the sensations to which they refer. A number of philosophers have thought that this presupposition is false. In this section I will comment briefly on four views about the justification of introspective beliefs that conflict with mine.

If we deny that beliefs about sensations can be confirmed by the sensations to which they refer, then it seems we must accept one of the following propositions: (1) beliefs about sensations are groundless – they are not justified by anything; (2) they are justified by other beliefs; (3) they are self-justifying; and (4) they are justified because they are produced by reliable cognitive mechanisms. Would we be well advised to accept one of these other views?

We find the most influential formulation of (1) in the writings of Wittgenstein. Here is Malcolm Budd's account of Wittgenstein's position:

> The question 'How does a person know when he can truly say that he is in pain?', where this question is asking for the *basis* of the person's assertions, is misplaced if the person knows what the word 'pain' means. His assertions lack any basis. . . . It follows that it is incorrect to maintain that the reason I have a right to be absolutely certain that I can truly say that I am in pain is that my remark has an absolutely secure basis, or that I have unshakeable evidence, or that I have an overwhelmingly good justification for what I say. My remark rests on nothing at all, in the sense that I have no reason that assures me of the probable or certain truth of my remark. My remark is ungrounded: in the self-ascription of pain I use the word 'pain' without a justification. . . .[11]

According to Wittgenstein, then, it would be wrong to say that one's beliefs about one's own sensations are justified by sensations, and it would also be wrong to say that they are self-justifying. (Perhaps Wittgenstein even held that there is something unhappy about the expression "beliefs about one's own sensations," but that is a different question.)

<hr>

11 See Malcolm Budd, "Wittgenstein on Sensuous Experiences" in Leslie Stevenson, Roger Squires, and John Haldane (eds.), *Mind, Causation, and Action* (Oxford: Basil Blackwell, 1986). The quoted passage occurs on p. 71.

131

Why did Wittgenstein hold this position? According to an interpretation that appears to be widely accepted, Wittgenstein was moved to adopt it by the perception that it makes no sense to speak of seeking evidence for the proposition that one is having a sensation of a certain kind, or of finding evidence for the proposition, or of assessing evidence for it. It makes no sense, for example, to speak of checking to see whether one has a pain, or of checking to see whether a sensation satisfies the condition that it must satisfy in order to count as a pain. There are no verification procedures associated with the concept of pain. Because this is true, there is no logical room for the claim that one can have evidence that one is in pain.

Perhaps this is just a caricature of Wittgenstein's reasoning. However, if it is an accurate account, then Wittgenstein was confused. According to the interpretation, Wittgenstein held that we have no method of obtaining evidence for beliefs about sensations, and also that we have no method of assessing such evidence. These observations are no doubt true, at least under some interpretations; but they have no tendency to show that beliefs about sensations are not supported by evidence. In order for a belief to be supported by evidence, it is enough for the evidence to be possessed by the believer and to stand in certain causal relations to the belief. It need not be true that the believer has found the evidence or that he or she has obtained it by applying some sort of verification procedure. Nor need it be true that the believer has assessed the evidence. Something counts as evidence by virtue of the role it plays in mediating between beliefs and the items to which the beliefs refer. It need not have been obtained in a certain way or have been subjected to a certain test.

There is a second way of reading Wittgenstein. He seems to have thought that it is impossible to be mistaken about one's own sensations, and he may have thought also that it is meaningless to describe the members of a category of beliefs as supported by evidence unless it is possible to be mistaken in holding beliefs that belong to the category. Together these two views lead to the conclusion that beliefs about one's own sensations cannot be supported by evidence. However, we have already seen that the first view is false: as we know from the previous section, it is wrong to claim infallibility for introspective beliefs. It is also true that the second view is badly in need of justification and defense.

At all events, quite apart from the fact that the arguments for Wittgenstein's position seem to be specious, it appears that the position is false. It seems plainly wrong to deny that beliefs about sensations can be justified. To deny this is to abandon all pretense of giving a philosophical account of justification which makes contact with our intuitions.

(2) is the view that beliefs about one's own sensations are justified by other beliefs. It is easy to underestimate this view; it seems prima facie to be obviously wrong. Thus, we normally think that if the justification of a belief derives from other beliefs, the latter beliefs must be antecedently held. But the course of one's sense experience can be highly unpredictable. (How could I have predicted a moment ago that there would be an itch in my left thigh at the present moment?) And if one's prior beliefs have not enabled one to anticipate one's current sensations, it seems they could not possibly provide a justification for the beliefs that register the existence and nature of those sensations.

When, however, one takes a deeper look, one finds that it is in fact possible to see one's beliefs as receiving their justification from inference. This is brought out quite clearly by an ingenious model of the justification of introspective beliefs that has been devised by Laurence BonJour.[12] In BonJour's model, the justification of a sensory belief does not depend entirely on beliefs that are antecedently held. Rather, the justification of a sensory belief depends in part on a metabelief that comes into existence either at the same time as or later than the given belief, and that classifies the given belief in terms of its provenience and its content. The rest of the justification is provided by a belief that *is* antecedently held. This second belief affirms the general reliability of beliefs that belong to the categories that are invoked by the metabelief. These two beliefs are seen as fitting together to form an argument of the following form:

> I have a cognitively spontaneous belief that Q, which is of kind K.
>
> Cognitively spontaneous beliefs of kind K are very likely to be true.
>
> Therefore, my belief that Q is very likely to be true.
>
> Therefore, (probably) Q.

(In describing the belief that Q as cognitively spontaneous, the first premise is making a claim about the origin of the belief: It asserts that the belief does not result from any "sort of deliberative or ratiocinative

12 See Laurence BonJour, *The Structure of Empirical Knowledge* (Cambridge, MA: Harvard University Press, 1985), section 6.5.

process, whether explicit or implicit," but rather occurs "in a manner which is both involuntary and quite coercive."[13] In describing the belief as a belief of kind K, the premise is simply classifying it as a sensory belief, or perhaps as a sensory belief that is concerned with a certain sense modality.) According to BonJour, a sensory belief is justified if it is possible to support it by embedding it in an argument such that (i) the argument has the given form, and (ii) the premises of the argument are themselves fully justified. Otherwise the belief is not justified.

Something like this picture is forced on us as soon as we decide to take (2) seriously. However, although I hasten to acknowledge that BonJour defends the picture with great subtlety and imagination, it seems to me that it is highly counterintuitive. As I see it, the model misrepresents the relevant epistemological relationships: According to intuition, first order beliefs about individual sensations are much more fundamental, epistemologically speaking, than general beliefs about the reliability of such first order beliefs. Moreover, it seems to me that one can be fully justified in holding a sensory belief even if, for one reason or another, one is unable to construct an argument of the indicated form. Thus, for example, extreme pain may temporarily render one incapable of the cognitive work that the construction of such an argument would require. (Think of your last horrible toothache.) Does someone in this situation lack justification for believing that he or she is in pain? Intuition counsels that the answer is "no."

This brings us to (3), which claims that beliefs about one's own sensations are self-justifying. It would take us too far afield to consider the positive arguments that have been constructed by defenders of this view. Instead I will simply state a couple of objections.

One problem with the view is that it is subject to counterexamples. Thus, it implies that beliefs about one's own sensations are always justified – or, more accurately, that they are justified unless they conflict with one's other beliefs. But it is easy to see that this implied proposition is false. Thus, for example, consider a situation in which S believes that he currently has an extremely faint pain in his left shoulder. Suppose that S does not actually have a pain in his shoulder, and that he holds the belief only because a thought-control device has been implanted in his brain. Suppose that he has not bothered to check up on the belief by focusing his attention on the area of phenomenal

13 BonJour, ibid., p. 117.

space that corresponds to his physical shoulder. Finally, suppose that the belief is fully compatible with his other beliefs. (3) implies that the belief is justified. But it is plain that this is wrong.[14]

There is also a deeper problem. This problem comes to the fore when we ask why it is that first-person beliefs about sensations have the special epistemic status that advocates of (3) mark by describing such beliefs as self-justifying. It is evident that there is a substantial epistemic difference between first-person ascriptions of sensations and third-person ascriptions, and it is also evident that epistemology is obliged to explain this difference. Now it seems that any explanation must appeal, sooner or later, to the fact that the relationship between first-person ascriptions and the sensations to which they refer is more intimate than the relationship between third-person ascriptions and the sensations to which *they* refer. Thus, it seems that it is necessary to say, sooner or later, that the special epistemic status of first-person ascriptions is due to the fact that they are related in a certain way to phenomena that are external to themselves. But if the epistemic status of first-person ascriptions is due to their relationships to phenomena that are external in this sense, it is misleading at best to describe such ascriptions as self-justifying. It is much more illuminating to say that they are justified by one or more aspects of these relationships.

Finally, we must consider (4) – the suggestion that beliefs about sensations are justified because they are produced by reliable mechanisms.

This suggestion is a special case of a more general view that has been defended with great subtlety in recent years by Alvin I. Goldman.[15]

14 There is an extremely insightful critical examination of (3) in a recent book by John L. Pollock. See his *Contemporary Theories of Knowledge* (Totowa, NJ: Rowman and Littlefield, 1986), 58–66. (The view about confirmation of beliefs by sensations that I develop in this chapter is, I believe, closely related to a position that Pollock defends (under the name "nondoxastic internalism") in this book. See, for example, p. 91. Like Pollock's view, my view is a form of foundationalism. However, unlike many foundationalists, I hold that introspective beliefs may need to receive a certain amount of warrant from other beliefs before they can count as *fully* justified. Indeed, I hold that this is true of even the most basic introspective beliefs, such as qualitative beliefs about pain. Although it is implicit in section IV, this last aspect of my position is largely ignored in this book. I hope to discuss it elsewhere.

15 See Alvin I. Goldman, "What is Justified Belief?" in G.S. Pappas (ed.), *Justification and Knowledge* (Dordrecht: D. Reidel, 1979), 1–23. For a more up-to-date presentation, see Goldman, "Strong and Weak Justification," *Philosophical Perspectives* 2 (1988): 51–69.

Very roughly speaking, Goldman holds that doxastic justification is always a matter of reliability. That is, where B is any belief, Goldman will say that B is justified if and only if B is the product of a reliable cognitive mechanism. Here, reliability is understood in terms of probability of truth: According to Goldman, a cognitive mechanism is reliable if and only if the beliefs that it produces are quite likely to be true.

I do not see how a reliabilist account of justification can possibly be correct. To my mind, the most damaging problem with such accounts is that they are incapable of explaining the appeal of skepticism.[16] If reliabilism were correct, then, to defend the thesis that we are not justified in holding our perceptual beliefs, the skeptic would have to argue that the mechanisms that produce our perceptual beliefs are unreliable. It follows that the skeptic would have to provide an enormous amount of empirical evidence concerning the success ratios of our cognitive mechanisms in the actual world. Perhaps it is true that some skeptics (for example, Sextus Empiricus) have thought it appropriate to proceed in this way; but mainstream skepticism – skepticism of the sort that one finds in Descartes's first *Meditation* – takes an entirely different direction. Instead of making empirical claims about the success ratios associated with our cognitive mechanisms in the actual world, mainstream skeptics offer arguments that are entirely a priori. (To see this, consider the version of Descartes's argument that is given in section I of the next chapter.) If reliabilist accounts of justification were correct, then a priori skeptical arguments would have no appeal whatsoever; for it would be clear to anyone who had acquired the concept of justification that the a priori premises of such arguments were irrelevant to the skeptic's conclusion, the claim that our perceptual beliefs are unjustified. However, as can be seen from their prominence in the history of

16 I hasten to add that this objection is not my only reason for rejecting reliabilism. Among other things, I also hold that reliabilism is incapable of handling, in a fully satisfactory way, counterexamples like the one that Goldman discusses in section III of "What is Justified Belief?" (op. cit., p. 188). That is, I doubt that the theory can accommodate cases in which beliefs are produced by reliable mechanisms but in which it is also true that the believers have evidence that calls their beliefs into question.

For another objection to reliabilism, see Stewart Cohen, "Justification and Truth," *Philosophical Studies* 46 (1984), 279–95. See also Thomas Senor, "Reliabilism and the Demon-World Objection," unpublished typescript, University of Arizona, 1987. (I believe that Cohen's objection is closely related to the objection that is raised in the text. However, they are not identical.)

philosophy, mainstream skeptical arguments are widely felt to be highly seductive.

VI

Up to now the discussion has involved a rather substantial idealization. I have written as if all cases of introspective awareness were uniform, but in fact there are salient differences. Introspective awareness involves belief, and to have a belief about something it is necessary to conceptualize it in some way. Thus, introspective awareness of sensations cannot be uniform unless it is true that all of our sensation concepts are pretty much alike in point of content. As we will see later on, however, these concepts are highly variegated. On the one hand, some concepts are purely qualitative, in the sense that one need only consult the immediate nature of sensations in determining whether to apply them. The concept of pain is a case in point. On the other hand, there are concepts whose contents derive entirely from the roles they play in an empirical theory (namely, folk psychology). Concepts that stand for certain types of visual sensations belong to this second category.

As I see it, there is a spectrum that runs from states of introspective awareness that involve purely qualitative concepts to states that involve highly theoretical concepts. Some of what I have said in this chapter is intended to apply to all points of this spectrum. For example, the analysis of basic awareness is intended to provide information about purely qualitative states of awareness and about highly theoretical states as well. No matter where on the spectrum it may occur, a state of introspective awareness involves a belief that is directed on a sensation, and the sensation is both the cause of the belief and the evidence by which it is confirmed. To be sure, there are differences in the degree of confirmation that introspective beliefs receive from sensations. But these differences are not visible from the level of abstraction on which the notion of basic awareness makes its home.

On the other hand, much of what I have said is intended to apply only to the states of awareness that lie at the qualitative end of the spectrum. This is especially true of the observations in section IV: the direct awareness thesis and the manifest nature thesis hold up pretty well when they are taken as observations about states at the qualitative end, but they are easily shown to be wrong when taken as observations

137

about other states. (See the discussion of awareness of visual sensations in Chapter 8.)

Thus, in this chapter I have been more concerned with qualitative awareness than with theoretical awareness. I will, however, have more to say about theoretical awareness in the context of a later discussion of concepts that stand for visual and auditory sensations.

6

Introspection and the skeptic

The claim that it is possible to obtain knowledge by sense perception has been a target for skepticism since the dawn of philosophy. In contrast, there have been no sustained skeptical challenges to our claim to be able to obtain knowledge by introspection. What accounts for the difference? Is it impossible to extend the arguments that have been formulated by skeptics so as to obtain new arguments that apply to introspective beliefs? If so, why? If one were to try to construct a skeptical argument concerning introspective beliefs, at exactly what points would one encounter problems?

I

It will be useful to begin by considering a line of thought that is frequently used to justify skepticism about sense perception. Let *PB* be the set of propositions that represent the perceptual beliefs of a certain normal subject, *S*. Further, let *SH* be the hypothesis that is obtained by conjoining the following five propositions: *S* is part of an elaborate psychology experiment that is being conducted in a laboratory on a remote planet; *S* is a brain in a vat; *S* is connected to a computer that monitors all of *S*'s thoughts; all of the sense experiences *S* has had up to now have been caused by events inside the computer; and in the future the computer will provide experiences like the ones that *S* has had in the past (that is, experiences that confirm the members of *PB* and that lead *S* to adopt new beliefs that are consistent with the members of *PB*). With these abbreviations in hand, we can summarize a standard skeptical argument as follows:

I am deeply indebted to Ivan Fox and to Sydney Shoemaker for inspiration, and to Joseph Levine for pointing out a mistake in an earlier version.

139

PB is logically incompatible with *SH*. $\qquad$ (1)

S is not justified in rejecting *SH*; for *S* is unable to rule *SH* out by adducing empirical evidence; and *S* is unable to bring forward any a priori arguments that count against it. $\qquad$ (2)

If *A* is a set of propositions and *q* is a proposition that is incompatible with *A*, then *x* cannot be said to be completely justified in believing the members of *A* unless *x* has grounds for ruling out *q*. $\qquad$ (3)

Hence, by (1), (2), and (3), *S* is not completely justified in believing the members of *PB* – even if the members of *PB* are in fact true in the actual world. $\qquad$ (4)

If *x* knows that a proposition is true, then *x* is completely justified in believing the proposition. $\qquad$ (5)

Hence, by (4) and (5), *S* cannot be said to know that the members of *PB* are true – even if they are in fact true in the actual world. $\qquad$ (6)

Although it seems prima facie that (2) must be wrong, skeptics have managed to argue convincingly that it should be accepted. Thus, they have pointed out that all empirical evidence is ultimately sensory in nature, and that there are no sense experiences that show that the members of *PB* are to be preferred to *SH*. (As can be seen by reflecting on its content, *SH* gives rise to exactly the same retrodictions and predictions about the realm of *S*'s sense experience as *PB*.) Moreover, when their opponents have tried to rule out hypotheses like *SH* by opposing arguments, skeptics have usually managed to come up with replies that are at least moderately convincing.

Now it is clear that there is no hope of using a line of thought that is fundamentally similar to (1)–(6) to justify skepticism about introspective beliefs. *SH* exploits the gap between the appearances on which our perceptual beliefs are based and the underlying reality to which the beliefs refer; *SH* would be incoherent if we could not hold appearances fixed while imagining changes in the underlying reality. It follows of course that there can be no counterpart of *SH* that applies to introspective beliefs. Thus, as the direct awareness thesis informs us, there is no gap between the entities on which our introspective beliefs are based and the entities to which they refer.

Perhaps, however, it is possible to construct a different sort of skeptical argument. When one peruses the contemporary literature on the mind–body problem, one sooner or later encounters the concept of *ersatz pain.*[1] Ersatz pain is described as an internal state that lacks qualitative character (that is, it does not count as a sensation), but that is equivalent to real pain in its causal relations to other internal states, to inputs, and to outputs. Like pain itself, it is said, ersatz pain occurs when there is bodily damage or the body is exposed to extremes of temperature or pressure. Moreover, ersatz pain can cause the same constellation of beliefs and desires as real pain, and it is therefore able to influence behavior in the same way. Now as Sydney Shoemaker has pointed out, there is a certain amount of tension between the view that one can be said to know that his or her actual pains are real pains and the view that it is logically possible for a human being to be in an internal state that satisfies the definition of ersatz pain.[2] Thus, suppose that it is logically possible for a human being to be in a state of this kind. Among other things, it follows that it is logically possible for a state other than real pain to cause S to remember the real pains that he has experienced in the past, and also that it is logically possible for a state other than real pain to cause S to think that his current state is qualitatively similar to the past experiences to which the memories in question refer. In view of these consequences, it is extremely tempting to conclude that it is logically possible for S to be in a state that he is incapable of distinguishing from real pain. But if this is true, how can S rule out the proposition that his actual state is a state of ersatz pain? And if S is unable to rule the proposition out, how can he claim to know that his actual state is a state of real pain?

Let us try to make the logical structure of this argument explicit. Let *RP* be the proposition that S is currently experiencing a real pain, and let *EPH* be the hypothesis that unbeknown to S an evil demon has recently replaced S's disposition to have real pains with a disposition to have ersatz pains.[3] (If you are a materialist, imagine that the transformation consists in the substitution of a bank of artificial neurons for a

---

1 See, for example, Ned Block, "Are Absent Qualia Impossible?", *The Philosophical Review* LXXXIX (1980): 257–74. In footnote 4, Block attributes the term "ersatz pain" to Larry Davis.

2 See Sydney Shoemaker, "Functionalism and Qualia," *Philosophical Studies* 27 (1975): 291–315. See also Shoemaker's "Absent Qualia are Impossible," *The Philosophical Review* XC (1981): 581–99. Both papers are reprinted in Shoemaker's *Identity, Cause, and Mind* (Cambridge: Cambridge University Press, 1984).

3 In addition to *EPH*, there is also the following more radical skeptical hypothesis: S has *never* had a disposition to have real pains, but has rather been disposed from birth to experience ersatz pains. As a result, unbeknown to S, his first-person ascriptions of pain have *always* been false.

bank of real neurons.) Finally, let us suppose that a skeptic puts forward the following argument:

RP is logically incompatible with *EPH*. (7)

S is not justified in rejecting *EPH*; for *S* is unable to rule *EPH* out on the basis of introspection, and *S* is unable to bring forward any a priori arguments that count against it. (8)

If p is a proposition and q is a proposition that is incompatible with p, then x cannot be said to be completely justified in believing p unless x has grounds for ruling out q. (9)

Hence, by (7), (8), and (9), *S* is not completely justified in believing *RP* – even if *RP* is in fact true in the actual world. (10)

If x knows that a proposition is true, then x is completely justified in believing the proposition. (11)

Hence, by (10) and (11), *S* cannot be said to know that *RP* is true – even if *RP* is in fact true in the actual world. (12)

According to our skeptic, this argument is sound. What about it? Is this claim correct?

Despite its being more radical, this second skeptical hypothesis can be ruled out by a line of thought that is in all essentials the same as the line of thought that I use later to rule out *EPH*. Moreover, it may well be that the more radical hypothesis is also vulnerable to a second objection. Specifically, it may be that it can be refuted by appealing to the account of the semantic properties of the concept of pain that is defended in Chapter 7. That account implies that the content of *S*'s beliefs about pain (including beliefs that are first-person ascriptions of pain) derives from indexical and/or causal relations between *S*'s concept of pain and the state to which *S* has applied that concept in the past. It follows that if *S* has always been disposed to experience ersatz pains, then his concept of pain stands for ersatz pain, not real pain. But if *S*'s concept of pain stands for ersatz pain, then, when *S* forms a belief to the effect that a current ersatz pain falls under his concept of pain, his belief must be true! Thus, if the semantic account of the concept of pain that is given in Chapter 7 is correct, and it is true that *S* has always been disposed to experience ersatz pain, then *S*'s first-person ascriptions of pain are really ascriptions of ersatz pain, and their truth values are therefore just the opposite of what the skeptic's hypothesis claims them to be.

This second point derives from an objection to skeptical arguments about perceptual knowledge that is due to Hilary Putnam. Perhaps the most interesting criticism of Putnamian objections is found in Anthony L. Brueckner, "Brains in a Vat," *The Journal of Philosophy* LXXXIII (1986): 148–67. I respond to Brueckner briefly in my review of Philip Pettit and John McDowell (eds.), *Subject, Thought, and Content* in *The Journal of Philosophy* LXXXVII (1990): 106–12.

II

Before giving the reply that seems to me to be right, I will comment briefly on four alternative replies.

(a) The first focuses on premise (9). According to (9), in order to be completely justified by a certain fund of evidence in believing that p, it must be true that one's fund of evidence gives one a sufficient reason to rule out all hypotheses that imply that it is false that p. (In short, it must be true that one's evidence *selectively confirms* the proposition that p.) This principle is of course closely related to premise (3) of the first argument. To use a name that has a certain currency in the literature on skepticism, we can say that (3) and (9) are members of the family of *counterpossibility principles*.

A number of philosophers have objected that counterpossibility principles are too strong. These philosophers acknowledge that one cannot be completely justified in believing that p unless one is in a position to rule out some of the hypotheses that are incompatible with p, but they deny that one must be in a position to rule out all such hypotheses. It is enough, they say, to be able to rule out all hypotheses that are *relevant alternatives* to p. Different members of this school explain the idea of a relevant alternative in different ways, so it is best to try to motivate the distinction between relevant and irrelevant alternatives by giving an example. Suppose you are inclined to believe that there is a squirrel on the road ahead of you. In order to be completely justified in holding this belief, the philosophers under discussion would say, you must have grounds for the belief that enable you to rule out the hypothesis that there is a small animal other than a squirrel on the road. However, it need not be the case that your grounds enable you to rule out the hypothesis that you are a brain in a vat who is being given misleading visual sensations by a computer that has been programmed to deceive you. The first alternative hypothesis is a relevant alternative, and the other one is not.[4]

Advocates of the relevant alternatives approach would presumably reply to skepticism about introspection in the same way they reply to

---

4 It seems that the relevant alternatives strategy made its first appearance in Fred Dretske's "Epistemic Operators" (*The Journal of Philosophy* LXVII (1970): 1007–23). For a comprehensive and illuminating critical study of this strategy, see Anthony L. Brueckner, "Skepticism and Epistemic Closure," *Philosophical Topics* XIII (1985): 89–117. See also Stewart Cohen, "How to Be a Fallibilist," *Philosophical Perspectives* 2 (1988): 91–123.

143

skepticism about sense perception. They would presumably say that *EPH* does not represent a relevant alternative to the proposition that *S* is in pain, and that *S* can therefore be completely justified in believing that he is in pain even if he is unable to rule *EPH* out.

Although the relevant alternatives approach can be made to seem fairly attractive, there is reason to think that we would be ignoring a crucial distinction if we were to use it as the foundation of our response to (7)–(12). I am strongly inclined to say that the skepticism represented by (7)–(12) is even more outrageously counterintuitive than the skepticism represented by (1)–(6). This is not to minimize the implausibility of (1)–(6). It is shocking. But, I think, (7)–(12) is even more shocking. An adequate answer to skepticism must acknowledge and explain this difference. It seems, however, that the relevant alternatives approach is incapable of meeting this challenge. It counsels us to respond to (1)–(6) by adding one or more qualifications to (3), and it counsels us to respond to (7)–(12) by adding similar qualifications to (9). At the very least, it seems that more should be said. Even if one thinks that (9) must be qualified, one should try to find another flaw in the skeptic's reasoning, a flaw that lies at a deeper level.

(b) The second reply is that *S* is entitled to reject *EPH* on the grounds that it is incoherent. By definition, ersatz pain has exactly the same functional properties as real pain. Accordingly, because real pain can cause *S* to form beliefs that involve *S*'s concept of real pain, the same must be true of ersatz pain. This shows that *S* would have to have a concept of real pain if *EPH* were true. But, the objection claims, it would not be appropriate to credit *S* with a concept of real pain in the circumstances in question. He would continue to use the words "real pain," and no doubt these words would express a concept. However, because he would have a firm disposition to apply this concept to ersatz pains and no tendency whatsoever to apply it to real pains, it is more appropriate to see the concept as a concept of ersatz pain than as a concept of real pain. (Remember that *S* would no longer be endowed with a disposition to have real pains if *EPH* were true.)

One could expand this line of thought by claiming that the concept of pain somehow contains or makes indexical reference to the disposition to have real pains. For example, one might claim that the content of the concept of pain can be represented by a description like "internal state that is a manifestation of *that* disposition." If this hypothesis were correct, then the intentional content of the concept of pain would change at the moment at which the demon played his wicked trick. The concept would automatically become a concept of ersatz pain.

Although I find this reply more plausible than its predecessor, I think that it is seriously flawed. It seems to me that on reflection we find ourselves obliged to reject the contention that the content of the concept of pain would change at the very moment when S's disposition to have pains was replaced with a disposition to have ersatz pains. We find that we should say instead that the content of the concept would survive the change for at least a short while.

Let us consider a similar question. Suppose that an evil demon removes McX's brain from his body at some point after McX has acquired the concept of a cow. Suppose also that the demon continues to send it stimuli by activating neural pathways that used to be attached to sense organs. Suppose finally that these stimuli cause McX to have sensations that represent an orderly continuation of his past experience. In these circumstances, McX would continue to believe true the sentence "There is a cow in front of me" when confronted with a cowish sensation. Would his term "cow" continue to denote cows? Or would it acquire a new denotation – would it perhaps come to denote whatever it is inside the demon that is ultimately responsible for McX's cowish sensations? Or would it cease to denote cows without acquiring a new denotation?

I am strongly inclined to answer that McX's term "cow" would retain its previous denotation for at least a short while. By the same token, I am strongly inclined to suppose that McX's concept of a cow would retain its intentional content for a certain period of time.

In general, it seems to me that the content of a kind-term or a kind-concept is not fixed entirely by one's dispositions to apply the term or concept to other things. Historical factors appear to play a role as well.

Because of these intuitions, I think it is a mistake to defend the charge that EPH is incoherent in the way we have been considering. It seems reasonable to suppose that the content of S's concept of pain would eventually change as a result of the demon's actions. But to establish that EPH is incoherent it would be necessary to show that it is logically impossible for there to be an internal state with the defining properties of ersatz pain, and to establish this it would be necessary to show that the content of the concept of pain could not survive the demon's actions even by a second. My view is that it is impossible to show this.

(c) The third reply is like the second in that it charges *EPH* with incoherence, but it defends the charge in a different way. It asserts that the intentional content of certain explicitly indexical beliefs depends on the capacity to experience pains, and that it is therefore impossible to continue to have beliefs of the sort in question after the capacity has been erased. Because the ability to produce such beliefs is one of the functional properties of pain, it follows that it is impossible for there to be a state other than pain itself that has the same functional role as pain.

Consider a case in which you have a pain and also a belief (inspired by the pain) that you would express by the sentence "Internal states of this type are abominable." It is clear that the content of this belief depends in part on the existence of the pain, and it is equally clear that your capacity to have beliefs of the same type as the given belief depends on the existence of your capacity to experience pain. But more: It is clear that pains play a major role in causing beliefs of this type. It follows that there is a functional property of pain that is not shared by internal states of any other sort.[5]

Although this objection appears to be sound, it does not pose a serious threat to skepticism. The skeptic can simply sidestep the objection by replacing *EPH* with a closely related hypothesis. Thus, instead of defining ersatz pain as a state that has exactly the same functional properties as real pain, he can define it as a state that is just like real pain in causal relations to all psychological states that are not explicitly indexical. He can then invite us to consider a hypothesis that is just like *EPH* except that it is based on this new definition of ersatz pain. It appears that this new hypothesis has all of the features of *EPH* that originally sparked the skeptic's interest. Moreover, it is free from debilitating logical and semantical flaws.

Because the skeptic has the option of replacing *EPH* with a similar hypothesis that is not incoherent, I propose to set the third reply aside. I will proceed as if *EPH* were fully coherent.

(d) Like the second and third replies, the fourth reply questions the coherence of *EPH*. However, instead of claiming that the intentional content of a concept or a belief depends on the capacity to experience pains, and that it is therefore impossible to preserve the concept or the

---

5 This is one way of putting a point made by Earl Conee in "The Possibility of Absent Qualia," *The Philosophical Review* XCIV (1985): 345–66. See especially pp. 354–56.

belief while erasing the capacity, it asserts that the qualitative character of pain is inextricably linked to the functional role of pain because the latter is definitive of the former. That is to say, the fourth reply defends the claim that it is logically impossible for there to be a state that lacks the qualitative character of pain but that possesses its functional role by asserting that the qualitative character of pain is identical with a congeries of functional characteristics.

The functionalist theory of qualitative states suffers from a number of problems. (See Chapter 3.) Those who are prepared to live with those problems will be able to use this fourth reply. A nonfunctionalist like me is obliged to look elsewhere.

In addition to the worries about (b)-(d) that I have already mentioned, there is the objection that they all fail to make contact with our gut-level intuitions about the skeptic's argument. When one first encounters *EPH*, one is inclined to say that one can see that it is false on the basis of introspective awareness. One is inclined to say that one is immediately aware of one's pains, and that in being aware of them one is aware of data that count decisively against *EPH*. In my case, at least, this intuition is extremely strong. However, (b)-(d) fail to take it into account. Indeed, in asserting that *EPH* is incoherent, they in effect claim that it is impossible for the data of experience to count against it.

III

What would have to be the case in order for *S* to be justified by introspection in rejecting *EPH*? It is natural to say that *S* is justified in rejecting *EPH* on introspective grounds if and only if *S* has introspective evidence that supports the proposition that *S* can still experience real pain. But what is it to have introspective evidence of this sort? The answer is obvious: One can be said to have introspective evidence for a proposition about one's sensations just in case one actually has sensations that confirm the proposition. It follows that *S* has evidence of the right sort if and only if he is currently experiencing real pain or he has experienced real pain in the recent past. Thus, it seems that *S* need not construct an argument in order to be justified by introspection in rejecting *EPH*. He need only be in a certain state. That is, he can overturn the skeptic's hypothesis by being in pain. (Here we find some possibly unexpected support for Aeschylus's contention that knowledge comes through suffering!)

It is evident that this line of thought calls the skeptic's position into question. The skeptic wants to claim that S is not justified by introspection in rejecting *EPH*. According to our current perspective, a defense of this claim should take the form of a proof that (despite S's beliefs to the contrary) S is not currently experiencing real pain and has not experienced real pain in the recent past. That is to say, in order to defend the claim the skeptic must try to establish an empirical proposition about S's state of mind. But to undertake this task is to abandon skepticism. The philosophical skeptic has no interest in establishing substantive propositions about the empirical world, but rather is concerned with normative questions about justification. It is the goal of the philosophical skeptic to show that we lack justification for certain of our substantive beliefs without taking a position on whether those beliefs are true or false.

It may be helpful to compare skepticism about introspective beliefs with one of the traditional forms of skepticism. Let us take another look at the situation involving *PB* and *SH*. The members of *PB* can be said to be confirmed by S's sense experiences, but it is arguable that the former are not selectively confirmed by the latter. It can seem that S's sense experiences have just as strong a tendency to confirm *SH* as to confirm the members of *PB*. In other words, it can seem that they are neutral between *SH* and the members of *PB*. Now this apparent neutrality gives the skeptic a right to maintain that S is not fully justified in believing the members of *PB* on the basis of sensory evidence. The skeptic can claim to have this right without denying that S has the sensory states that common sense attributes to him, and without trying to show that the members of *PB* are false. On the other hand, the situation involving *EPH* is quite different. It cannot be argued with any plausibility that S's sensory evidence is neutral between his introspective beliefs and *EPH*. If S is currently experiencing pain, he has evidence that confirms his belief that he is in pain. By the same token, he has evidence that shows (decisively) that *EPH* is false. Hence, in order to claim that S is not fully justified in believing that he is in pain, the skeptic must argue that this belief is not confirmed by sensory evidence. That is to say, he must deny that S is currently experiencing pain. But this is not what the skeptic wants to do. Qua philosophical skeptic, he is concerned to establish a purely conditional claim – namely, the claim that even if S is in pain, he is not completely justified in believing that he is in pain.

IV

At this point, our skeptic might protest that we have reached a conclusion that is unfavorable to him only because we stacked the deck at the outset by accepting an excessively liberal answer to the question of what should count as a refutation of *EPH*. He might urge that it is not enough that S possess sensory evidence that strongly and selectively confirms the proposition that he is in pain. In addition, the skeptic might say, S must be capable of distinguishing between situations in which he has such evidence and situations in which he does not.

In effect, then, the skeptic is proposing that there are two conditions that one must satisfy in order to be completely justified in believing that p. First, there is the condition that is expressed by the second counterpossibility principle. According to this condition, in order for it to be true that one is completely justified in believing that p on the basis of a certain fund of evidence, one's evidence must selectively confirm (and strongly confirm) the proposition that p. Second, there is the following *discernibility condition*: In order to be completely justified in believing that p on the basis of evidence of type ϕ, one must be able to distinguish between situations in which one has evidence of type ϕ and situations in which one lacks such evidence.

Prima facie, at least, it seems that if the skeptic can defend the discernibility condition, he will be in a position to conclude that S is not completely justified in believing that he is in pain. For the following proposition is prima facie correct:

> S is incapable of distinguishing between situations in which he is in pain and situations in which he is in ersatz pain. (13)

And (13) implies that S is not always capable of distinguishing between situations in which he has introspective evidence that he is in pain and situations in which he lacks such evidence. To be sure, it may be that the intuitions that cause us to favor (13) are misleading. However, as is shown by the prominence that (13) enjoys in the literature, these intuitions are strong and widely shared. Someone who wishes to reject (13) must shoulder the burden of proof.

Is it reasonable to accept the discernibility condition? If it is to serve the skeptic's purposes, the condition must be interpreted in such a way that it entails (14).

149

One is not completely justified in believing that *p* unless it is true that, for every situation σ in which one lacks evidence that *p*, if σ were actual, one would be able to recognize that one was in a situation in which one lacked evidence that *p*. (14)

Nothing weaker will do. This is because the skeptic's purposes will not be served unless *S* fails to satisfy the discernibility condition. *S* fails to satisfy the requirement that (14) imposes, but he would satisfy a less general requirement (provided that the lack of generality was not due to restrictions that were entirely ad hoc). After all, *S* has no problem in recognizing that he is not in pain in normal situations. It is only in *outré* situations like the one described by *EPH* that his ability to recognize that he is not in pain breaks down.

(14) is extremely strong – much stronger than the counterpossibility principles that we encountered earlier. It is, I think, obvious that it is too strong to be acceptable. Take, for example, someone who is now taking a bath in the actual world. Let us suppose that this individual's cognitive mechanisms are in good working order and that at the present moment he is fully conscious. Now, even though all is well with our bather in the actual world, we must recognize that there are possible situations in which he lacks evidence that he is taking a bath but in which he is unable to recognize that he lacks it because Alzheimer's disease has erased the concepts that such recognition requires. Equally, there are possible situations in which he lacks evidence of the kind in question but is incapable of recognizing that he lacks it because he is unconscious (or dead). If (14) were correct, the existence of possible situations of these sorts would prevent us from saying that our bather has evidence in the actual situation that completely justifies him in believing that he is taking a bath. But this is absurd. The fact that one's cognitive mechanisms are undetectably impaired in some other possible situation has no tendency to show that one's beliefs are not justified in the actual situation.

Is it really true that nothing weaker than (14) will do? What if the skeptic tries to reformulate (14) by restricting the variable "σ" to exclude situations in which one is either unconscious or not in possession of one's faculties? Is there no way of doing this that is not ad hoc? In particular, what about (15)?

One is not completely justified in believing that *p* unless it is true that, for every situation σ in which one lacks evidence that *p and in which one's*

150

cognitive faculties are in good working order, if σ were actual, one would be able to recognize that one was in a situation in which one lacked evidence that *p*. (15)

(15) is immune to counterexamples involving unconscious subjects and also to counterexamples involving subjects who suffer from Alzheimer's disease. Moreover, there is no justification for describing the italicized condition as ad hoc. Still, there is a problem. It appears that (15) allows us to say that S is completely justified in believing that he is in pain. This is because the new restriction on "σ" excludes situations in which *EPH* is true. Situations in which *EPH* is true could not possibly count as situations in which S's cognitive faculties are in good working order, for they are situations in which a crucial component of S's cognitive faculties – his capacity to acquire sensory evidence of a certain kind – has been destroyed, and in which, as a result, he has a stable disposition to misclassify certain of his internal states. Certainly we would have to say that S has suffered a cognitive impairment if he were to lose a capacity to reach true beliefs about internal states as a result of losing a capacity that has a genetically determined function within his cognitive system. Hence, even though it is true that S would be unable to recognize *EPH*-situations if they were actual, it is impossible to get a result that would be useful to the skeptic by combining this fact with (15).

This argument stands or falls with the claim that situations in which *EPH* is true do not count as situations in which S's cognitive faculties are in good working order. The main justification for this claim derives from a doctrine that was defended in the previous chapter. As we saw there, when a subject introspectively recognizes a sensation as a case of pain, the sensation is playing a dual role. It is the object of a state of awareness, but it is also the epistemic foundation of the state of awareness, in the sense that it confirms or justifies the belief on which the state of awareness is based. Now if pains provide the epistemic foundation for states of awareness of pain, and this arrangement is determined by genetic factors, we must say that the ability to feel pain is an essential constituent of the cognitive mechanism that sustains introspective awareness of pain. But this implies that someone who has been deprived of the ability to feel pain has undergone a cognitive impairment. And of course this last proposition implies in turn that situations in which *EPH* is true do not count as situations in which S's cognitive faculties are in good working order.

V

It is important to distinguish between the discernibility condition and another principle that it superficially resembles. According to this other principle (hereafter called the *weak exclusion principle*), in order to be completely justified in believing that p on the basis of evidence of type ϕ, one must be in a position to exclude (that is, to rule out) all hypotheses that imply that one is not in possession of evidence of type ϕ. The principle may also be formulated as follows: In order to be completely justified in believing that p on the basis of evidence of type ϕ, one must be able to determine whether or not one has evidence of type ϕ. As this second formulation shows, it is easy to confuse the weak exclusion principle with the discernibility condition. However, careful scrutiny reveals that the two principles are quite different. The weak exclusion principle is a claim about one's actual epistemic state: It says that one must be able to use one's actual cognitive faculties and the information that is actually available to one to rule out the members of a certain set of hypotheses. On the other hand, when it is interpreted in such a way that it can be seen to imply (14), the discernibility condition claims that one must be capable of certain epistemic achievements in other possible situations – including possible situations in which one's cognitive faculties are quite different than they are in the actual situation.

Although there are philosophers who maintain that it is too strong, to my mind the weak exclusion principle is quite appealing. Because of its similarity to the discernibility condition, those of us who find the weak exclusion principle appealing will often be tempted to embrace the skeptic's position. However, we can now see that it would be a mistake to allow this similarity to influence us. The similarity is only skin deep.

It is easy to see that S does in fact satisfy the weak exclusion principle in the case we have been considering. In the case at hand, the relevant proposition is the proposition that S has a pain, and the relevant evidence is one of S's current pains. Thus, in the case at hand, the weak exclusion principle comes to this: In order to be completely justified in believing that he has a pain on the basis of evidence that consists in his having a pain, S must be in a position to exclude all hypotheses that imply that S does not have a pain. Now we have already seen that S satisfies the relevant counterpossibility principle: He has evidence that strongly and selectively confirms the proposition that he has a pain.

152

Because this evidence selectively confirms the proposition in question, S is able to rule out all conflicting propositions. But this means that he is able to rule out all hypotheses that imply that he does not have a pain. So he satisfies the weak exclusion principle by virtue of satisfying the second counterpossibility principle. Q.E.D.

It is not always true that someone who satisfies the latter requirement will also satisfy the former. Quite the contrary. This holds in the present case only because the proposition that S believes is identical with the proposition that describes his evidence for the belief. (That is to say, the proposition that is the value of "p" in the weak exclusion principle in the present case is identical with the proposition that is the value of "one has evidence of type ϕ.")

Here the skeptic may protest that we have once again failed to do justice to his position. He may acknowledge that the weak exclusion principle fails to support his skeptical claims, but maintain that we are committed to a stronger principle that serves his purposes quite nicely. This new principle is the *strong exclusion principle*:

> In order to be completely justified in believing that p on the basis of evidence of type ϕ, one must be in a position to exclude all hypotheses that imply that one is not in possession of evidence of type ϕ, and one must be in the position by virtue of having grounds other than the forementioned evidence of type ϕ.

The strong exclusion principle tells us that S cannot claim to be justified in believing that he is in pain unless he satisfies the following requirement: S is able to rule *EPH* out, and he is able to rule it out on grounds other than his current pain. This requirement is of course much harder to satisfy than the corresponding requirement that derives from the weak exclusion principle. Indeed, it is easy to see why the skeptic might think that it *cannot* be satisfied.

Fortunately, the skeptic's contention to the contrary notwithstanding, it is quite clear that we are not committed to the strong exclusion principle. It is much too strong to command our assent. Unlike the weak exclusion principle and the various members of the counterpossibility family, which are supported by intuitions and which seem – prima facie, at least – to be entirely benign, it is obvious from the outset that this new principle puts justification and knowledge out of our reach. Interpreted in the way that the skeptic intends, the principle implies that where g_1 is any ground on which a belief is based, one must have some other ground g_2 that supports the proposition that one has g_1.

That is to say, it implies that justification inevitably involves an infinite regress. Thus, to think that our ordinary concept of justification commits us to the strong exclusion principle is to suppose that it transparently requires us to do the impossible. And this supposition is patently absurd. What inducement could Mother Nature possibly have for endowing us with a concept of justification that has this feature? Or, assuming that our concept of justification owes more to our creative powers than to our genetic inheritance, what inducement could we possibly have for devising such a concept? And if we had devised one, what inducement could possibly lead us to retain it?

VI

It appears that Sydney Shoemaker was the first philosopher to investigate the possibility of constructing a skeptical argument concerning introspective knowledge. However, instead of endorsing skepticism, Shoemaker in effect transformed a skeptical argument into a defense of functionalism. He retained the premises of the argument but supplemented them by taking the denial of the conclusion as a new premise. He then pointed out that this slightly richer set of premises supports the functionalist's view that the functional role of pain is definitive of its qualitative character. In this section I will offer an assessment of Shoemaker's line of thought.

The first premise of Shoemaker's argument is (16).[6]

> If ersatz pain is possible, the presence or absence of the qualitative character of pain would make no difference to its causal consequences that would make it possible for anyone to distinguish cases of genuine pain from cases of ersatz pain. (16)

Shoemaker doesn't make the other premises fully explicit, but given his endorsement of (16) it is easy to see that the rest of his argument goes like this:

> If the presence or absence of the qualitative character of pain would make no difference to its causal consequences that would make it possible for anyone to distinguish cases of genuine pain from cases of ersatz pain, no one is ever completely justified in believing on the basis of introspection that he or she is in pain. (17)

6 See Shoemaker, *Identity, Cause, and Mind* (Cambridge: Cambridge University Press, 1984), p. 316.

If no one is ever completely justified in believing on the basis of introspection that he or she is in pain, no one can be said to know on the basis of introspection that he or she is in pain. (18)

One often does know on the basis of introspection that he or she is in pain. (19)

Hence, ersatz pain is impossible. (20)

(20) supports functionalism because it implies that the qualitative character of pain is internally related to its functional role.

(19) is of course the denial of the skeptic's conclusion. Shoemaker does not offer a justification for it. Perhaps he feels that the falsity of the skeptic's conclusion is self-evident.

I urge the reader to join me in rejecting (17). Premise (17) stands or falls with the following more general claim: One cannot be completely justified in believing that one is in pain unless one can distinguish between situations in which one has evidence that one is in pain and situations in which one lacks such evidence. But this claim is a special case of the discernibility condition, and it manifestly suffers from the flaw that we observed in considering the latter. It is much too strong to be acceptable.

Like the discernibility condition, (17) enjoys a certain specious plausibility by virtue of its superficial similarity to a principle that commands our respect. Thus, it can seem that (17) says no more than this: One cannot be completely justified in believing that one is in pain unless one can rule out the hypothesis that one is in ersatz pain. This claim is a special case of the weak exclusion principle. It appears to be correct.

If Shoemaker could replace (17) with the new claim, he would be on firm ground. However, if he were to replace (17) with the new claim, it would be necessary to replace (16) with the following stronger proposition: If ersatz pain is possible, someone who is in pain is incapable of ruling out the hypothesis that he or she is in ersatz pain. And our line of thought in section III implies that this stronger proposition is false. (As we saw in section III, someone who is in pain has evidence that selectively confirms the proposition that he or she is in pain. And, of course, if one has evidence that selectively confirms a proposition, one is in a position to reject all propositions that imply that the given proposition is false.)

PART FOUR

Sensory concepts

7

Concepts of bodily sensations: Their semantic properties

In recent years, philosophers have been much concerned with questions about the contents or meanings of the sensation concepts that we employ in everyday life. They have presented and defended a wide variety of positions. At one end of the spectrum is the view that our sensation concepts acquire their contents from internal ostensive definitions, and that these concepts are therefore purely phenomenological, in the sense that the question of whether a given concept applies to a given sensation depends entirely on the immediate phenomenological nature of the sensation. At the other end of the spectrum we find the view that our concepts of sensations are similar in content to theoretical concepts such as the concept of gravity and the concept of electric charge. According to this second view, the contents of our sensation concepts derive from the roles that the concepts play in our common-sense theory of mental activity. This view denies that the question of whether a concept applies to a given sensation has anything to do with the immediate phenomenological nature of the sensation. To determine whether the concept applies to a sensation, the view maintains, it is necessary and sufficient to consider the causal role that the sensation plays in the internal economy of the being in whom it occurs. If the sensation bears the right causal and counterfactual relations to other things (namely, to external stimuli, to behavior, and to other internal states), it falls under the concept. Otherwise it does not.

Questions about the contents of sensation concepts have important connections with metaphysical questions about the nature of the sensations for which these concepts stand. Indeed, the question of whether we will be able to accept type materialism depends to a large extent on our disposition of these other questions. Consider for a moment the second of the two views of which we have just taken note. If, as this

I have been helped immensely by a number of conversations with Sydney Shoemaker.

159

view contends, it is part of our concept of a certain type of sensation that sensations of that type play a certain causal role, then the causal role in question will be constitutive of what it is to be a sensation of that type. But if this is true, it will not be possible to identify the type of sensation with a type of neurological state. For the nature of a neurological state depends entirely on the properties of its constituent neurons and on the relations they bear to one another, not on the causal and counterfactual relations that the state bears to other things. It seems, then, that the second view is incompatible with type materialism. But then, insofar as we are moved by the considerations that seem to favor type materialism, we are under an obligation to criticize the second view and to defend an alternative account of contents.

It is also true that questions about the contents of our concepts are intertwined with some of the main questions about the epistemological status of introspective beliefs. Consider the second view again. It claims that the contents in question derive largely from assumptions about the relations between types of internal states, types of external stimuli, and types of behavior. This claim implies that our concepts of sensations are theoretical – that when one subsumes a sensation under one of our everyday sensation concepts, one is making a move that is more or less on a par, epistemologically speaking, with the move one makes when one attributes a certain mass to a remote star or a certain rate of growth to the economy of a nation. But if the move of subsuming a sensation under one of our everyday concepts is theoretical, then the qualified Cartesian picture of introspective beliefs that I recommended earlier can hardly be correct. For that picture represents our introspective beliefs as having a degree of accuracy and a degree of stability that theoretical beliefs could not possibly possess.

For both metaphysical and epistemological reasons, then, it would be useful to have an adequate account of the semantic properties of our sensation concepts. I will give such an account in this chapter. In sections I and II I will focus on concepts of the following three kinds: concepts that stand for highly circumscribed types of bodily sensations (for example, the concept of pain, the concept of the sensation of heat), concepts that stand for highly circumscribed types of gustatory sensations (for example, the concept of the taste of lemons), and concepts that stand for highly circumscribed types of olfactory sensations (for example, the concept of the olfactory sensation associated with the smell of frying bacon). Section III is concerned with concepts that stand for less highly circumscribed types of sensations – that is, with generic concepts like the concept of a gustatory sensation and the concept of an olfactory sensation. I will also discuss the most highly generic sensation concept of all – the concept of a sensation itself.

I will be primarily concerned to convince the reader that our sensation concepts are highly variegated, both in the sense that the set of all sensation concepts is highly heterogeneous, and also in the sense that each sensation concept exemplifies a set of semantic properties that is rather disparate. Theories that offer uniform accounts of the semantic properties of sensation concepts tend to be grotesque oversimplifications. To have a chance of success, a theory must be a hybrid whose genetic material derives in part from the functionalist tradition and in part from the introspectionist tradition.

Although I will say a number of things about the semantic theories that other writers have offered, my discussion will be limited to theories that represent sensation concepts as factual or descriptive. I will say nothing about theories that imply that the content of first-person ascriptions of sensations is largely expressive. These theories, which derive ultimately from Wittgenstein, conflict with the intuition that first-person ascriptions of sensations can be literally true and literally false. In this book this intuition has the status of a nonnegotiable constraint on theories of content.

I

The reader may well feel skeptical as to whether the concepts to be considered in this section and the next have a unifying common nature. After all, we will be considering a class that includes the concept of pain, the concept of an itch, the concept of a sensation of pressure, the concept of a sensation of heat, the concept of the taste of lemons, and the concept of the olfactory sensation associated with frying bacon. Is there really a feature that is shared by all of these concepts? If so, what is it?

The reason for grouping these rather heterogeneous concepts together is this: It is clear that each of them has what might be called an *infralinguistic* dimension. Or perhaps, for the sake of clarity, we should say that each of them is in effect a pair of concepts, and that every pair has one member that is infralinguistic. Consider pain, for example. One of the concepts that stands for pain is linguistic: It can be identified with the ability to use the term "pain" correctly in internal and external discourse. But there is also an infralinguistic concept of pain.

161

This follows from two observations that seem incontestable. First, it is impossible to have propositional attitudes (expectations, beliefs, desires, fears, and so on) about something unless one has a concept that stands for that thing. And second, organisms often have propositional attitudes toward their bodily sensations without having mastered a language. (Small children may be said to expect to feel pain in certain circumstances, to fear pain, to desire certain pleasures, and so on. Similar things may be said of chimpanzees and other higher animals.)

Although "infralinguistic" is the term I shall use, it would in some ways be more informative to describe the concepts in question as "infratheoretical." One is able to acquire and to apply the concepts without having mastered a theory of any kind, and in particular, without having acquired the information about the functional properties of sensations that is contained in folk psychology. This is because infralinguistic concepts of sensations are purely qualitative, in the sense that the question of whether a given sensation falls under a concept of this sort is determined purely by the qualitative character of the sensation. When an adult attends to a pain, he or she typically thinks of it in terms of its immediate qualitative nature. The same is true when an adult expects to feel a pain or desires that a pain cease. In general, adults tend to think of pain as a certain sort of feeling, not as a state with such-and-such representational content or as a state with such-and-such causes and effects. It seems reasonable to suppose that the same is true of small children and animals. A small child can attend to a pain – or expect a pain or desire that a pain cease – without thinking of it as something that has a representational property or a causal role.

Our purpose here does not require us to form an opinion as to whether infralinguistic sensation concepts are innate or acquired, but we do need to observe that they seem to arise spontaneously. That is to say, it seems likely that they are among the earliest concepts to enter our conceptual vocabulary, and this makes it seem unlikely that they are introduced by reference-fixing or by ostensive definition, or by any other process that requires semantic sophistication. Rather they come into existence and acquire their contents by processes that are largely subpersonal and involuntary.

As I see it, we have infralinguistic concepts of all our bodily sensations, and the same is true of our concepts of olfactory and gustatory sensations. Small children can look forward to pleasurable tastes and to feelings of warmth before they have attained a theoretical perspective on such sensations. Moreover, we make daily use of infralinguistic concepts even as adults. When, as an adult, one identifies a taste or an olfactory sensation, one does not do so by taking note of its functional properties. Rather one identifies it by recognizing its purely qualitative characteristics. Appreciation of functional properties comes about as a result of this qualitative identification. (Recall that you can be aware of a certain taste, and even recognize it as familiar, while being unable – for the moment, at least – to identify it as a taste *of* retsina or as a taste *of* absinthe, or as a taste *of* some other kind.)

Before leaving the topic of infralinguistic concepts, we should briefly consider the following question: By virtue of what fact or facts is it true that infralinguistic sensation concepts stand for such properties as *being a pain* and *being an itch*? After all, there are other properties that might be thought to be equally good candidates. Suppose that p is a pain that is possessed by a certain individual i. p is an instance of *being a pain*, but it is also an instance of *being a pain possessed by i*. And if i is a Rotarian, then p is an instance of *being a pain possessed by a Rotarian*. Further, it is an instance of *being a pain or a gerbil*. By virtue of what fact or facts is it true that i has an infralinguistic concept that stands for *being a pain* rather than one of these other properties?

This is a complex and difficult question. I will not attempt to give a fully satisfactory answer here. However, part of the answer is surely that there are nomological relations between certain mental states that involve the concept of pain (that is, certain fundamental beliefs and desires) and the property *being a pain*. Thus, for example, instances of *being a pain* can cause one to believe that one is in pain, and they have this capacity by virtue of the fact that they are instances of this property. On the other hand, there are no nomological relations between the mental states in question and the property *being a pain possessed by i*, nor between the states in question and either the property *being a pain possessed by a Rotarian* or the property *being a pain or a gerbil*. Unlike *being a pain*, which is a universal, these other properties are incapable of playing a role in laws of nature. (Suppose i has a pain, and that this pain causes i to believe that he is in pain. The pain cannot be said to cause the belief by virtue of being an instance of *being a pain possessed by i*. Nor by virtue of being an instance of *being a pain possessed by a Rotarian*. Nor by virtue of being an instance of *being a pain or a gerbil*. It has its causal powers solely by virtue of being an instance of *being a pain* (and other universals).)

II

What about our *linguistic* concepts of such sensations as pains and itches? What is the correct theory of the contents of these concepts? Or, equivalently, what is the correct theory of meaning for terms like "pain" and "itch"? Before sketching the answer that I prefer to these questions, I will discuss several alternative answers. I hope that the problems confronting alternative theories will help to motivate the theory that I wish to recommend.

1. *Externalist* theories of meaning claim that names for bodily sensations like pain are equivalent with descriptions that pick the sensations out by invoking their typical external causes or their typical external effects (or both their typical external causes and their typical external effects). For example, an externalist theory might claim that "pain" is equivalent to "the internal state that is normally caused by damage to the body and by bodily disturbances that threaten to produce such damage." But what is meant by "equivalence" here? Externalism can take two rather different forms, and the forms are distinguished by their answers to this question. According to one form, names for sensations are equivalent with descriptions in the sense of being synonymous with them. I believe that this form received its earliest and its most convincing formulations in the writings of Smart and Armstrong. The second form, which was first sketched in an extremely rich and interesting paper by Michael Levin, maintains that descriptions are used to fix the reference of names of sensations.[1] As I understand them, both forms of externalism have implications that are highly counterintuitive. Where P is a commonsense sensation term, I understand both forms to be committed to the proposition that one would normally appeal to causal and counterfactual relations to extramental phenomena in justifying a first-person ascription of P.[2] But nothing could be

---

1 For the first form, see J.J.C. Smart, "Sensations and Brain Processes," *The Philosophical Review* LXVIII (1959): 141–56, and D.M. Armstrong, *A Materialist Theory of the Mind* (New York: Humanities Press, 1968). For the second, see Michael E. Levin, "Kripke's Argument against the Identity Thesis," *The Journal of Philosophy* LXXII (1975) :149–67.

2 In general, where P is a psychological term, if a theory claims that users of P fix its reference by a certain description, D, I take the theory to be committed to the proposition that the properties mentioned by D are the properties to which one would normally appeal in justifying an ascription of P (in the way in which, for example, one would normally appeal to the property *being the brightest heavenly body in the western sky immediately after sunset* in justifying an ascription of "Hesperus").

164

farther from the truth! It is transparent that our best and most fundamental test for whether something belongs to the extension of "pain" is direct and immediate. To apply our best and most fundamental test, it suffices to consult the qualitative nature of a sensation. There is no need to take its causal relations to external phenomena into account. Indeed, there is no need to take account of any of its relations to any other phenomena.

2. As we saw earlier, analytic functionalism claims that every name in our commonsense psychological vocabulary is synonymous with a folk-psychological description (that is, a description based in a certain way on the laws of folk psychology). As we also saw, this claim implies that each such name refers to a functional property, where a functional property is a property of internal state-tokens such that the tokens that exemplify the property do so by virtue of their causal and counterfactual relations to other internal state-tokens, to external stimuli, and to behavioral phenomena.

We should refresh our memories of the technical content of these ideas here. To this end, let us suppose that $T_1, \ldots, T_u$ is a list of our everyday names for psychological state-types, that FP is the conjunction of some set of axioms that represents a systematization of folk psychology, and that $FP(X_1, \ldots, X_u)$ is the formula that results from replacing $T_1, \ldots, T_u$ with the property variables $X_1, \ldots, X_u$ in FP. With these conventions in hand, we can say that a Ramsey functional description is a description of the form "being a state-token y such that it is possible to find state-types $X_1, \ldots, X_u$ such that (1) FP $(X_1, \ldots, X_u)$ and (2) y exemplifies X_i."[3] The psychological names $T_1, \ldots, T_u$ correspond in a systematic way to the descriptions that have this form: T_1 corresponds to the description that has the variable X_1 in clause (2); T_2 corresponds to the description that has the variable X_2 in clause (2); and so on. Exploiting this correspondence, we can express the central doctrine of analytic functionalism as follows: Each term T_i is synonymous with the corresponding Ramsey functional description.

In assessing analytic functionalism we took note of three objections, each of which appears to give us a sufficient reason for concluding that

---

3 Descriptions of this form are equivalent to terms that look like this: "The property ϕ such that, necessarily, ϕ is exemplified by a state-token y if and only if it is possible to find state-types $X_1, \ldots, X_u$ that satisfy these two conditions: (1) $FP(X_1, \ldots, X_u)$, and (2) y exemplifies X_i."

165

analytic functionalism is on the wrong track.[4] These objections suggest certain criteria of adequacy that should guide the search for a better theory. It will be useful to make these criteria explicit here.

First, as the absent qualia argument shows, a theory of meaning for sensation terms should not entail that the question of whether a being has sensations can be answered solely on the basis of information about the functional organization of the being. Any theory that carries this entailment can be refuted by counterexamples involving Blockean androids. Second, as the absent role argument shows, a theory should not entail that a being must have a functional organization of any particular sort in order to be capable of having sensations. It appears to be a fact that sensations can occur in beings that differ greatly from one another in point of functional organization. A theory of meaning for sensation terms must accommodate this fact. Third, a theory should not entail that we cannot be fully justified in making first-person ascriptions of sensation terms until we have taken the causal and counterfactual properties of our internal states into account. The question of how such ascriptions are justified is complex, and there may be no one answer that holds in all cases. (See Chapter 8.) However, it seems clear that in at least some cases (for example, the case of "pain"), the question of whether one is justified in ascribing a sensation term to one of one's own internal states depends only on the immediate qualitative nature of the state. A theory of meaning must explain this.

There is also a fourth criterion that is suggested by our study of functionalism – though this time the point is one that emerged in the course of our reflections on psychofunctionalism. It seems to be the case that we would be willing to attribute sensations to Blockean androids if we believed that our own brains were composed of homunculi. This point suggests that our intuitions about the distribution of sensations are fundamentally anthropocentric – that our intuitions as to whether other beings have sensations are influenced by our perceptions concerning the nonfunctional similarities between the other beings and ourselves. A theory of meaning for sensations must analyze this anthropocentricity and provide an explanation of it.

It turns out to be rather difficult to satisfy these criteria of adequacy. Analytic functionalism fails to satisfy any of them, and most of the other theories of meaning that are known to me fail to satisfy at least one. The only exception is the theory that I will begin to develop after

4 See Chapter 3, section III.

166

we have taken a look at one more inadequate theory, a theory I call *synthetic folk psychologism*.

3. Unlike analytic functionalism, which asserts that commonsense sensation terms have the same meanings as folk psychological descriptions, synthetic folk psychologism contends that such descriptions are used to fix the reference of commonsense sensation terms. To be more specific, synthetic folk psychologism distinguishes between sensation terms that count intuitively as descriptions and sensation terms that count intuitively as names. ("Sensation of heat" falls in the first group, because it seems to be a truncated form of a description like "the sensation-type that is normally caused by heat." "Pain" falls in the second group, as does "sensation" itself.) Synthetic folk psychologism claims that the reference of commonsense names for sensations is fixed by folk psychological descriptions.[5]

The goal of synthetic folk psychologism is to provide a theory of meaning that preserves what it regards as our main intuition about the problem of other minds. As we saw, if analytic functionalism is true, the claim that certain androids have sensations follows immediately from the proposition that they can exemplify state-types that realize certain of the functional roles determined by folk psychology. Synthetic folk psychologism is concerned to accommodate an intuition that is incompatible with this result. This intuition can be expressed as follows: Although I have the right to be pretty confident that other human beings have sensations, I should be extremely skeptical about ascriptions of sensations to androids, even when the androids are functionally isomorphic to human beings.

It might be useful here to remind ourselves of the distinction between a functional role and a functional property. A property χ is a functional role if and only if (1) χ is a second-order property that is exemplifiable by internal state-types, and (2) every internal state-type

---

5 As far as I know, synthetic folk psychologism is not widely held. The earliest source appears to be Levin, op. cit., where, however, it is not sharply distinguished from the second of the two forms of externalism that I mentioned here. Apart from Levin's paper, I know of only five published discussions of the view: Sydney Shoemaker, "Functionalism and Qualia," *Philosophical Studies* 27 (1975): 291–315; William G. Lycan, "Psychological Laws," *Philosophical Topics* 12 (1981): 9–38 (see especially footnote 10); Henry Jacoby, "Eliminativism, Meaning, and Qualitative States," *Philosophical Studies* 47 (1985): 257–70; Earl Conee, "The Possibility of Absent Qualia," *The Philosophical Review* XCIV (1985): 345–66 (see footnote 32); and William G. Lycan, *Consciousness* (Cambridge, MA: Bradford Books, 1987), pp. 10, 20–21, and 134 (footnotes 18 and 19).

that exemplifies χ does so by virtue of its nomological relations to other internal state-types, to types of external stimuli, and to types of behavioral phenomena. As we saw, every functional role is associated with a unique functional property. Thus, where χ is a functional role, there is the property of exemplifying some state-type or other that exemplifies χ. This is the functional property associated with χ. It is a first-order property in the sense that it is exemplified by concrete events rather than state-types.

Where P is a name that belongs to our commonsense psychological vocabulary, analytic functionalism maintains that P refers to a functional property. Suppose the claim is that P refers to ϕ. Now ϕ corresponds to a certain functional role – say, χ. Instead of claiming that P refers to ϕ, synthetic folk psychologism asserts that it refers to ψ, where ψ is the state-type that occupies the functional role χ in members of the species homo sapiens. Thus, according to synthetic folk psychologism, we confer meaning on "pain" by saying that it is to refer to the state-type that plays such-and-such functional role (hereafter role F) in human beings. The qualification "in human beings" is needed as a hedge against the possibility that different state-types play role F in different kinds of beings. Without the qualification, we would have a description (namely, "the state-type that plays role F") that might well suffer from indeterminacy of reference.

Synthetic folk psychologism contends that we confer meaning on "pain" by saying that it is to refer to the state-type that plays role F in human beings. But this contention can be understood in two ways. It can be understood as the claim that our use of "pain" is such as to make it synonymous with the description "the state-type that plays role F in human beings." Or it can be taken to mean that we use this description to fix the reference of pain. The second interpretation is the one that synthetic folk psychologism intends. Some terms for sensations seem intuitively to have the status of names, and "pain" is a paradigm case. Synthetic folk psychologism tries to preserve this intuition by denying that terms like "pain" are synonymous with descriptions. It claims that such terms are intimately related to descriptions, but it analyzes this relationship in terms of the notion of reference-fixing, not in terms of synonymy.

According to synthetic folk psychologism, then, "pain" refers rigidly to the state-type that plays role F in human beings in the actual world. Synthetic folk psychologism does not claim that there are any essential connections between this state-type and role *F*. It is compatible with the intuition that the state-type plays quite different functional roles in other possible worlds, and also with the intuition that there are possible worlds in which it plays no role at all.[6]

It should be emphasized that this doctrine has no tendency to imply that it is a mistake to use terms like "pain" in describing the internal states of members of other species, nor even that it would be a mistake to use them in describing the internal states of androids. The fact that, for example, the referent of "pain" is exemplified by tokens that are found in human beings has no tendency to imply the view that the referent of "pain" is not exemplified by tokens that are found in badgers or in beings like C4PO. (It is compatible with this view, but it does not imply the view.) Moreover, even if we could show conclusively that the physical state-types associated with human beings are entirely disjoint from the physical state-types that are associated with badgers or beings like C4PO, it could still be true that the referent of "pain" is exemplified by badger-tokens and C4PO-tokens. This is because the description that fixes the reference of "pain" leaves it open whether the referent is physical or nonphysical. Synthetic folk psychologism is compatible with a dualistic account of pain and other sensory states, and it is also compatible with a materialistic account.

Synthetic folk psychologism is in many ways a more appealing doctrine than analytic functionalism, but it nonetheless suffers from two serious shortcomings. First, it is too narrow: It offers an account of the semantic properties of the commonsense terms for sensations that count as names, but it has virtually nothing to say about the commonsense terms that count as descriptions. Second, because synthetic folk

---

6 By "state-type" I mean "universal." Thus, I see synthetic folk psychologism as making use, either explicitly or implicitly, of the concept of a universal in fixing the reference of commonsense sensation names.

   As I see it, synthetic folk psychologism should claim that we use descriptions of the following form (or equivalent descriptions) to fix the reference of sensation-terms: "The property ψ such that ψ is a universal and ψ exemplifies the functional role F in human beings." I see descriptions of this form as nonrigid designators: When used in talking about the actual world they pick out the universals that play the appropriate functional roles in actual human beings, and when used in modal contexts they pick out the universals that play the appropriate functional roles in the beings that are members of homo sapiens in other possible worlds. Of course, terms like "pain" can be rigid designators even if the descriptions used to fix their reference are nonrigid.

psychologism maintains that we fix the reference of "pain" by a description that invokes a functional role, it is committed to the view that we normally justify claims to the effect that a subject is in pain by appealing to the fact that he or she is in a state that has the right sort of cause and the right sort of effects.[7] This is no doubt exactly right when taken as a thesis about what one does in justifying claims about the pains of others, but it is hopelessly wrong when taken as a thesis about what it is that justifies first-person ascriptions of "pain." First-person ascriptions are justified by the qualitative natures of the ascriber's internal state. One sees that something is a pain by seeing that it hurts, not by taking an inventory of its causal relations.

4. According to a fourth view, expressions like "pain" belong to the same category as such expressions as "water," "lemon," and "tiger." They are *natural kind words*: They stand for universals that play a role in the laws of nature that obtain in the actual world. The author who has written most illuminatingly about natural kind words is Hilary Putnam. I will briefly summarize his views about terms for nonpsychological kinds, and then I will offer a suggestion as to how those views might be applied to terms like "pain."

The conceptual basis of Putnam's theory consists of four notions: the notion of a syntactic marker, the notion of a semantic marker, the notion of a stereotype, and the notion of an extension. Roughly speaking, a syntactic marker is just a concept that stands for a logicogrammatical category: The concept of a noun is a syntactic marker, as are the concepts of an adjective and a verb. A semantic marker is a high-level concept that represents one of the fundamental categories in our commonsense classificatory system. Where F is a term, the concept expressed by a term G is one of the semantic markers associated with F if the sentence "All F's are G's" is analytic. In other words, the semantic markers associated with a term are supposed to explain the analyticity of certain of the classificatory judgments that involve the term. Putnam tells us that the concept expressed by "animal" is a semantic marker, and that the same is true of the concepts expressed by "living thing," "artifact," and "period of time." A stereotype is

a standardized description of features of the kind that are typical, or 'normal', or at any rate stereotypical. The central features of the stereotype generally are *criteria* – features which in normal situations constitute ways of recognizing if a thing belongs to the kind or, at least, necessary conditions (or probabilistic necessary conditions) for membership in the kind. Not all criteria used by the linguistic community as a collective body are included in the stereotype, and in some cases the stereotypes may be quite weak. Thus (unless I am a very atypical speaker), the stereotype of an elm is just that of a common deciduous tree. These features are indeed necessary conditions for membership in the kind (I mean 'necessary' in a loose sense; I don't think 'elm trees are deciduous' is *analytic*), but they fall far short of constituting a way of recognizing elms. On the other hand, the stereotype of a tiger does enable one to recognize tigers (unless they are albino, or some other atypical circumstance is present), and the stereotype of a lemon generally enables one to recognize lemons. In the extreme case, the stereotype may be *just* the marker: the stereotype of molybdenum might be *just* that molybdenum is a *metal*.[8]

Finally, there is the notion of an extension. The use Putnam makes of this notion is much the same as the use made of it by other authors: The extension of a term of divided reference (for example, "lemon") is a class of individual substances or individual events, and the extension of a mass term (for example, "water") is the fusion or logical sum of all of the parts of reality that count as portions of some type of stuff. Whether the extension of a term is a class or a fusion, it is composed of all and only those entities to which the term can be correctly applied.

Once Putnam has these notions in hand, he is in a position to formulate the core doctrines of his theory. He writes:

> My proposal is that the normal form description of the meaning of a word should be a finite sequence, or 'vector', whose components should certainly include the following (it might be desirable to have other types of components as well): (1) the syntactic markers that apply to the word, e.g. 'noun'; (2) the semantic markers that apply to the word, e.g. 'animal', 'period of time'; (3) a description of the additional features of the stereotype, if any; (4) a description of the extension. . . .
>
> Thus the normal form description for 'water' might be, in part:

8 See Hilary Putnam, "The Meaning of 'Meaning'" in Putnam's *Mind, Language and Reality* (Cambridge: Cambridge University Press, 1975), 215–71. The quoted passage occurs on p. 230.

SYNTACTIC MARKERS	SEMANTIC MARKERS	STEREOTYPE	EXTENSION
mass noun, concrete;	*natural kind; liquid;*	*colorless; transparent; tasteless; thirst-quenching; etc.*	H_2O *(give or take impurities).*[9]

But this proposal about the normal form of descriptions of meaning is only one of his main doctrines. Another one is the view that the first three components of a semantic vector represent the competence of a mature speaker: They represent the specifically linguistic knowledge that guides the speaker's use of a term. And the third main doctrine is the claim that the first three components of a semantic vector do not uniquely determine the fourth component. The extension of a term is not uniquely determined by what the speaker knows in knowing how to use the term.

What is it, then, that does determine the extension of a term? Putnam tells us that the extension of a natural kind term is determined in one of two ways. (He thinks that other terms are like kind terms in this respect, but this additional thesis need not be considered here.) In some cases, he says, a kind term can be said to have a certain class (or fusion) as its extension because (1) the class (or fusion) consists of the components of reality that exemplify some natural kind, and (2) the users of the term have a history of applying the term to components of reality that are members of the class (parts of the fusion) and not to other things. Thus, according to Putnam, if there are entities in other parts of the universe that have all of the properties that are included in the stereotype of lemons, but that differ from lemons at the microlevel in such a way as to count as exemplifications of a different natural kind, they do not belong to the extension of "lemon." In other cases, the extension of a term is fixed by the classificatory dispositions of a group of individuals who are seen as experts by the other members of their linguistic community. This happens when the normal members of a linguistic community believe that they are incapable of distinguishing between components of reality that are included in the extension and components that are not, and they are therefore willing to defer to experts on questions about the application of the term.

9 See Putnam, ibid., 269.

Assuming that "pain" is a natural kind word, what should Putnam say about it? I suggest that he should claim that the vector for "pain" looks roughly like this[10]:

SYNTACTIC MARKERS	SEMANTIC MARKERS	STEREOTYPE	EXTENSION
count noun, concrete	*natural kind, sensation;*	*being an internal state of a type that is normally caused by damage to the body or by extremes of pressure or temperature; being a state of a type that normally causes organisms to seek to end the condition that causes the state; being a pain;*	*the class of individual pains.*

There are two features of this vector that make it seem prima facie to be rather non-Putnamian, but actually there is a Putnamian rationale for both of them. In the first place, because the property, *being a pain* uniquely determines the class of individual pains, and because this property is included in the stereotype, we must conclude that the stereotype uniquely determines the extension. This means that the vector is an exception to one of Putnam's main doctrines. However, given Putnam's account of stereotypes, it seems entirely appropriate to assign *being a pain* to the stereotype in this case; for it is clear that this property is a criterion that guides us in determining whether or not to apply "pain" to individual sensations. Assuming that "pain" is a kind term, if Putnam wishes to maintain his definition of the notion of a stereotype, he should acknowledge that there are exceptions to his claim about the relationship between stereotypes and extensions. Second, the stereotype is redundant. Because *being a pain* uniquely determines the extension of "pain," there is a sense in which the other components are unnecessary. Nevertheless, it seems appropriate to

10 Henry Jacoby has offered a vector-based account of "itch" that is in some ways similar to my vector for "pain." See Jacoby, op. cit., 265.

include these other properties for the same reason that it seems appropriate to include *being a pain*. Stereotypes consist of the properties on which we rely most heavily in deciding whether to apply terms or to refrain from applying them. One relies almost exclusively on *being a pain* in deciding whether to apply "pain" to one's own sensations, but the situation is quite different in other cases. In deciding whether to apply it to the sensations of others one relies exclusively on the other components of the stereotype.

I am strongly inclined to think that our vector gives a satisfactory account of the semantic properties of "pain." Moreover, I think it is possible to devise vectors for several other sensation terms (for example, "itch") that are equally good. But I also think that the prospects of this approach are quite limited, for it seems to me that "pain" is not at all typical of sensation words. "Pain" is a name. Further, "pain" is a rigid designator: If ψ is the state-type to which it refers in the actual world, then it refers to ψ even in worlds in which ψ has a rather different functional role, and indeed, even in worlds in which ψ cannot be said to have a functional role at all. Other sensation terms tend to lack these properties. First, most sensation terms are not names in any sense, but are rather abbreviations of causal descriptions. Consider "the sensation of heat," "the taste of lemons," and "the olfactory sensation corresponding to the odor of frying bacon." It is clear, I think, that the first of these is roughly synonymous with "the sensation-type that is produced by heat in normal human observers in normal perceptual situations," that the second is roughly synonymous with "the taste-type that is produced by lemons in normal human observers in normal perceptual situations," and that the third is roughly synonymous with "the olfactory sensation-type that is produced by the odor of frying bacon in normal human observers in normal perceptual situations." Second, it is pretty clear that, for example, "the sensation of heat" undergoes a reference-shift in certain other possible worlds. Consider a world which is like the actual world except that in it human beings tend to undergo a functional inversion at some point in midlife. As a result of this inversion the state-types that they initially call "the sensation of heat" and "the sensation of cold" come to exchange certain aspects of their functional roles. Specifically, the state-type that is produced by heat comes to be produced by cold, and the state-type that is initially produced by cold comes to be produced by heat. It is clear, I think, that after accommodating to the change a denizen of this world will use "the sensation of heat" to refer to the state-type whose tokens represent heat in his new circumstances. To do otherwise would be to ignore the constraints that are imposed on use by the *meaning* of "the sensation of heat." (If pain and itching were to exchange functional roles, one might very well decide to use "pain" to refer to the new occupant of the functional role of pain. But this move would be dictated by the need to communicate effectively with other speakers, not by the meaning of "pain.")

Because expressions like "the sensation of heat" refer to different state-types in different worlds, it would be a mistake to try to describe their semantic properties by vectors like the one given here. The foregoing vector assigns only one referent to "pain," the implication being that "pain" refers to the same state-type in all possible worlds. What we need for expressions like "the sensation of heat" is an account that specifies the pattern according to which they take on new referents in new worlds.

5. At the beginning of this section we resolved to investigate a rather heterogeneous class of expressions that includes terms for highly circumscribed types of bodily sensations (for example, "pain," "the sensation of heat"), terms for highly circumscribed types of gustatory sensations (for example, "the taste of lemons"), and terms for highly circumscribed types of olfactory sensations (for example, "the gustatory sensation corresponding to frying bacon"). We saw three paragraphs ago that Putnamian vectors seem to provide an adequate theory of meaning for a subset of this class – namely, the terms that count as names for highly circumscribed types of bodily sensations. It is time now to try to decide on an account for the remaining members of the class.

The remaining members are for the most part what I will call *basic descriptions*. A basic description has two components, the first of which is either a highly generic general term (typically "sensation" itself), or a general term from an intermediate level of genericness (for example, "olfactory sensation"). The second component of a basic description is typically a prepositional phrase (for example, "of heat") or a participial phrase (for example, "corresponding to frying bacon"), the point of which is to place a restriction on the scope of the first component.

Thus, our topic here is the question, "What are the semantic properties of basic descriptions?" However, instead of considering this question in its most general form, let us focus on the special case of it that involves "the sensation of heat." This expression seems to be sufficiently typical that our conclusions about it will apply to other basic descriptions as well.

I wish to recommend a theory of the semantic properties of "the sensation of heat" that I will call the *dual criterion theory*. This theory consists of three claims. First, it asserts that "the sensation of heat" is more or less synonymous with the causal description "the state type ψ such that (1), necessarily, ψ is exemplified only by sensations, and (2) tokens of ψ that occur in normal human beings in normal perceptual circumstances are caused to occur by heat." Second, the dual criterion theory claims that the state-type that satisfies (1) and (2) in the actual world is a certain qualitatively individuated characteristic with which we are all introspectively acquainted. Third, the theory claims that we are guided by two different criteria in determining whether to apply "sensation of heat" to a particular concrete event. If the event is an internal state-token that belongs to someone else, one applies a criterion that is directly authorized by (1) and (2). Specifically, one tries to determine whether the token fulfills the conditions that we use to fix the reference of "sensation" (these turn out to be largely external – see the account of "sensation" in the next section), and to determine whether the token is caused by heat. On the other hand, if the event is an internal state-token of one's own, one applies a criterion that is not directly authorized by (1) and (2). Specifically, one uses introspection to determine whether the token exmplifies the qualitative characteristic ψ, where ψ is the characteristic that happens to be produced by heat in the actual world.

We should feel entirely comfortable about this third claim, for it merely invites us to see our use of "sensation of heat" as an instance of a familiar pattern. It frequently happens that we are guided in ascribing an expression by a criterion that is not directly authorized by the content of the expression. Consider "the first husband of Leslie." Suppose that an individual named "David" is the referent of this description, and that those who have an interest in talking about Leslie's former husband are able to recognize David by his physical appearance. Suppose finally that a friend of Leslie's, Priscilla, is in the middle of giving a thumbnail sketch of Leslie to a newcomer. Priscilla sees David approaching and says "See, there's Leslie's first husband." This is an ascription of the description. In making this ascription, Priscilla is only aware of the physical appearance of David. Of course, she has a longstanding belief to the effect that the person with the appearance in question is the first husband of Leslie, but this belief does not come before her mind. She moves directly from her perception of David to the ascription.

The third claim presupposes that we have a capacity, which is entirely independent of language, for recognizing instances of the qualitatively individuated state-type that is normally produced by heat. But we have already found reason to believe that we have infralinguistic concepts of all of the basic types of bodily sensations. Once we have determined that one of these concepts stands for the same sensation-type as the expression "the sensation of heat," we are capable of recognizing that "sensation of heat" can be applied to an individual sensation without checking to see that the sensation has the appropriate causal and counterfactual characteristics.

Some might worry that the dual criterion theory is incompatible with intuitions about the contingency of functional roles. Most of us would agree that, for example, it is possible for there to be a world in which the following sentence is true: The sensation of heat is nomologically correlated with cold rather than heat, and the sensation of cold is nomologically correlated with heat rather than cold. Because the dual criterion theory asserts that "the sensation of heat" is more or less synonymous with the description "the sensation-type that is nomologically correlated with heat," it can seem that this sentence would be contradictory if the dual criterion theory were true. By the same token, it can seem that the dual criterion theory is clearly wrong.

To block this objection it is sufficient to observe that a description can interact with a modal context in two different ways. Consider the description "the biggest fish in the sea," and suppose that it refers to Jones when it appears in nonmodal contexts. Further, consider the sentence "It could be the case that the biggest fish in the sea is a tuna." Let us agree to interpret the initial modal operator as expressing alethic rather than epistemic possibility. Even after we have fixed the sense of the modal operator by this agreement, the sentence is ambiguous. Understood in one way, it is true if there is a possible world w such that whatever it is in w that has the property expressed by "biggest fish in the sea" also has the property expressed by "tuna." That is to say, understood in one way, it is true if there is something in w – perhaps Jones, perhaps something else – that uniquely possesses both of these two properties. On the other hand, it can also be understood as a claim about Jones. Construed in this second way, it is true if there is a world w such that the being who possesses the first property in the actual world (Jones) possesses the second property in w. (Note that this truth-condition can be fulfilled in w even if Jones does not have the first property in w.)

In other words, descriptions are more flexible than names. Questions of ambiguity aside, a name can be used in only one way: It is always used to refer to the same entity, whether the context is modal or not. We might say that a name is strictly rigid. On the other hand, it would be wrong to say that a description is strictly nonrigid. Depending on the intentions of the user, a description can be used as a nonrigid designator, and it can also be used to refer rigidly to the entity to which it refers in the actual world.

Like other descriptions, "the sensation of heat" can be put to two different uses. When it is used nonrigidly, the sentence "The sensation of heat is nomologically correlated with cold rather than heat" expresses a contradiction. However, it can also be used as a rigid designator, and when it is, the statement expressed by this sentence is not contradictory. The statement is false in our world but true in other worlds.

III

In this section I will sketch and defend a view about the semantic properties of sensation-concepts that have a higher degree of genericness than the ones we have considered thus far. I will begin by offering an account of the properties of the most highly generic sensation concept of all – the concept of a sensation itself. I will then discuss the family of concepts that consists of such moderately generic notions as the concept of an olfactory sensation.

When embarking on an examination of the concept of a sensation, it is a good idea to begin by taking a look at the property for which the concept stands. For *being a sensation* is quite different than the qualitative characteristics under discussion in the previous section. Where ϕ is a qualitative characteristic that exhibits a fairly low degree of genericness (for example, *being a pain*), it will be found that all instances of ϕ resemble one another in qualitative character. But this is not true of instances of *being a sensation*. This property is exemplified by the current pain in my left leg and by the gustatory sensation that is currently being produced by the cherry Lifesaver in my mouth. These sensations are completely different in qualitative character – the difference between them is as great as the difference between a falling leaf and a wolf howling at the moon. To be sure, it is clear that the sensations have *something* in common. It is obvious that they share a number of functional properties, and that these functional properties are also exemplified by all of the other sensations that are owned by human beings. Further, it seems reasonable to suppose that all human sensations will be seen to resemble one another in intrinsic characteristics when it becomes possible to view them from the perspective of a mature neurology. The point is just that instances of *being a sensation* do not always resemble one another in a respect that is accessible to introspection.

In reply to this, it might be said that all sensations are qualitatively similar to one another, at least in an ancestral sense of "similar," in that they all exemplify the characteristic *having a location in phenomenal space*. This answer has a certain appeal. After all, if we count positions in the visual field and positions in the auditory field as phenomenal locations, it seems correct to say that all normal human sensations have the characteristic. Indeed, it can seem to be impossible to conceive of a sensation that is not in phenomenal space. To see this, focus your attention on a pain and try to conceive of something that is just like it except that it has no positional characteristic. You may feel that trying to do this is like trying to conceive of a house that does not have a determinate shape.

I think, however, that there are grounds for resisting the appeal of this reply. When one thinks about it, it comes to seem rather likely that there are lower organisms that are capable of having sensations but lack the capacity to endow them with positional qualities. Certainly an organism could find it useful to know that its body had encountered a dangerous level of temperature even if it was incapable of determining what part of its body was in greatest danger. This would be useful because it could respond by trying to get all of its body to a cooler place.[11] Further, even if there are no such organisms in the actual

---

11 There are occasional references to unlocated sensations in actual human subjects in the clinical literature. Thus:

> The sensory cortex is not concerned primarily with the recognition of crude sensory modalities, such as pain, thermal sense, and mere contact. These apparently enter consciousness at the level of the thalamus, and their appreciation is retained even after complete destruction of the sensory area. "The sensory activity of the cortex . . . endows sensation with three discriminative faculties. These are: (1) recognition of spatial relations, (2) a graduated response to stimuli of different intensity, (3) appreciation of similarity and difference in external objects brought into contact with the surface of the body." (Head, 20). . . . In severe lesions the patient, although aware of the stimulus and its sensory modality, is unable to locate accurately the point touched. . . .

This passage is from Raymond Truex and Malcolm Carpenter, *Human Neuroanatomy*, 7th edition (Baltimore: Williams and Wilkins, 1977), 565–66.

I am indebted to Ivan Fox for this reference and also for a stimulating and helpful conversation about unlocated sensations.

world, it seems reasonable to suppose that they are nomologically possible.

But isn't there a problem here? I acknowledged a while back that it can seem impossible to conceive of a sensation that has no location in phenomenal space, and I am claiming now that it is nomologically possible for there to be locationless sensations. Isn't there a certain amount of tension between these views?

I think it may well be true that if it is impossible to conceive of its being the case that p, it isn't nomologically possible that p. (Even though conceivability is not an adequate positive test for nomological possibility, it is arguable that inconceivability is an adequate test for nomological *im*possibility.) Thus, to preserve the consistency of my position, I must claim that despite appearances to the contrary, it is possible to conceive of an unlocated sensation. And in fact, I think that this claim is defensible. As Sydney Shoemaker has pointed out to me, the impression that it is impossible to conceive of an unlocated sensation can be explained away by distinguishing between conceiving and imagining, and by supposing that we have a tendency to confuse the two. It seems possible to conceive of an unlocated sensation – it seems that we just did so in thinking of an organism that is incapable of endowing sensations of heat with positional qualities. However, we are incapable of imagining an unlocated sensation. (This follows from three observations: First, to imagine a sensation of a certain kind is to form a sensory image of a sensation of that kind; second, our ability to form sensory images of sensations is limited by our ability to have sensations; and third, we human beings are incapable – in normal circumstances, at least – of having sensations that lack positional qualities.) Accordingly, unless we take pains to distinguish between conceivng that p and imagining that p, we are in danger of coming to hold that unlocated sensations are inconceivable.

I am inclined to think, then, that there is no purely qualitative similarity relation that is both fully accessible to introspection and universal, in the sense of linking sensations from all modalities. What is the significance of this conclusion? In the first place, the conclusion allows us to rule out the conjecture that the concept of a sensation acquires its content from an internal ostensive definition. Internal ostension presupposes similarity relations that are introspectively determinable. Second, the conclusion shows that it would be a mistake to postulate a qualitative infralinguistic concept that stands for the characteristic *being a sensation*. If we are incapable of seeing on the basis of introspection that all instances of *being a sensation* are similar in their qualitative natures, it cannot be true that we have a concept that groups instances of this property together on the basis of qualitative resemblance. And if we lack a concept that groups instances together on the basis of qualitative resemblance, we cannot be said to have a purely qualitative concept of the property.

Turning now to the question of what should be said about the *term* "sensation," I would like to recommend the view that we fix the reference of this term by a folk-psychological description – specifically, by a description of the form "the state-type that plays such-and-such functional role in human beings." The distinctive features of this proposal are motivated by some of the considerations that came to our attention earlier. Thus, it is necessary to include the qualification "in human beings" in order to protect the proposal from one of the main charges against analytic functionalism – the complaint that it commits us to saying that androids can have sensations. And it is necessary to invoke the notion of reference-fixing rather than the notion of synonymy because "sensation" is strictly rigid: It is always used to refer to the same entity, whether the context is nonmodal or modal.

This cannot be the whole story. After all, we are able to determine that "sensation" can be ascribed to some internal state-tokens and not to others on the basis of introspection alone. There is no need to check to see whether a token meets the conditions associated with some folk-psychological description. But how can this be? Given that we do not have a purely qualitative concept for the property *being a sensation*, how can we recognize that "sensation" is applicable to an internal state-token by unaided introspection? The answer, I think, is that we do not use a single, highly generic concept to determine whether it is appropriate to apply "sensation" to a state-token, but rather a group of concepts that have a comparatively low degree of genericness. Specifically, we rely on a purely qualitative concept that stands for pain, a purely qualitative concept that stands for the property determined by "the sensation of heat," and other concepts of the same sort.

As I see it, then, we should embrace an account of "sensation" that postulates two rather different criteria for applying the term. According to this view, we use a folk-psychological description to fix the reference of "sensation," and we are guided by the functional properties expressed by this description in applying the term to the internal states of others.[12] But we are capable of seeing that these functional properties are realized by qualitatively individuated state-types such as the one that serves as the referent of "the sensation of heat." When we do see this we form a disposition to be guided by the state-types in making first-person ascriptions of "sensation."

Given that our use of "sensation" is guided by a qualitative criterion as well as a functional criterion, it might seem to be misleading to claim that we appeal to functional characteristics in fixing the reference of the term. The claim seems to imply that the functional criterion is more fundamental than the qualitative criterion, and one might think that this implication is unfortunate. In fact, however, the functional criterion deserves its position of prominence. Apart from the fact that they realize many of the same functional characteristics, the qualitative characteristics of sensations have very little in common that is accessible from the perspective of common sense. It is only because we are aware of the common core of their functional roles that we think of them as being characteristics of the same kind. By the same token, it is only because we are aware of the common core of their functional roles that we find it natural and important to group their instances together under a single rubric – to apply the same term to pains, to sensations of heat, to sensations of pressure, to sensations of taste, and so on. It follows that the functional criterion is internally related to our reason

12 To be more precise: We fix the reference of "sensation" by a description of the form "the property ψ such that ψ is a universal and ψ realizes the functional role F in human beings." Here "F" abbreviates a description of the sort mentioned in footnote 3 – that is, a description based on the Ramsey sentence of a set of axioms for folk psychology.

Although it takes all of folk psychology to specify the functional role to which we appeal in fixing the reference (as can be seen from the fact that all of the axioms of folk psychology are constituents of the Ramsey sentence that occurs in the reference-fixing description), there are some parts of folk psychology that are more directly relevant to specifying that role than others.

What are the most important things that folk psychology tells us about this role? One of the most important things is surely this: If ψ is a state-type that occupies the role, instances of ψ carry information about extramental states of affairs that are of interest to the beings to whom the instances belong, and they play a certain characteristic role in the causation and confirmation of beliefs that refer to these extramental states of affairs. Here is another important fact about the role: If ψ is a state-type that occupies the role, instances of ψ tend to carry their information in a special form – a "qualitative" form that can be partially captured by saying that the mode of representation associated with sensations is quite different than the mode associated with propositional representations such as beliefs and sentences. (For an interesting attempt to analyze this difference, see Fred I. Dretske, *Knowledge and the Flow of Information* (Cambridge, MA: Bradford, 1981, 136–38.)

for having a term that is as highly generic as "sensation." This is not true of the qualitative criterion.

Is there any reason to prefer this account of "sensation" to an account modeled on the Putnamian theory of "pain" that we considered earlier? It seems that if we were to devise a Putnamian vector for "sensation," it would have to be so different from the foregoing vector for "pain" that it would be misleading to say that the former was modeled on the latter. Given that the characteristic *being a pain* is included in the stereotype for "pain," the nonqualitative properties that appear in the stereotype are in a certain sense redundant. The extension of "pain" is fully determined by the qualitative component of the stereotype, and the qualitative component provides an adequate basis for explaining why it is natural and important to group all of the members of the extension together under a single rubric. It follows that there is no need to give a full description of the functional role of pain in specifying the stereotype; it suffices to list a few properties of external stimuli and of behavioral phenomena that are fairly reliable signs of the existence of pain. The situation is quite different in the case of "sensation." In specifying a stereotype for this second term it would be necessary to give a full description of the functional role of *being a sensation*, for otherwise the stereotype would not provide a basis for explaining why it is natural and important for us to have a term with an extension that is as broad as that of "sensation." It would be necessary to use a full functional description (that is, a description that incorporates the Ramsey sentence for some complete axiomatization of folk psychology) in specifying a stereotype, and it would be necessary to add the information that we use this description in fixing the reference of "sensation." It follows that if we were to give a Putnamian account of the semantic properties of "sensation," the account would have to be virtually identical to the account I have been recommending. It would certainly have to be quite different in form from the account of "pain" that I recommended earlier.

So much for the semantic properties of the term "sensation." What about the properties of terms from the middle level of genericness? Or, to reduce this question to a more manageable form, what about the semantic properties of "olfactory sensation"? The answer that seems to me to be right is closely related to the dual criterion theory.

First, it seems intuitively correct to say that "olfactory sensation" picks out a type of sensation by implicitly referring to the phenomena that are the normal extramental causes of sensations of that type. To be more specific, it seems correct to say that the term refers implicitly to stimuli that produce sensations by acting on our odor-detecting sense organs. Accordingly, it seems that something like the following must be right: "Olfactory sensation" is synonymous with "sensation of the type ψ such that (1) ψ is nomologically connected with types of stimuli that act on the nostrils, and (2) ψ is not nomologically connected with types of stimuli that act on sense receptors of other kinds."[13]

Second, it seems that we are able to determine whether "olfactory sensation" is applicable to a sensation on the basis of unsupplemented introspection. This means, I think, that at some point early in our use of the term we come to realize that there is an introspectible characteristic (hereafter called "α") that fulfills the conditions expressed by (1) and (2) in the foregoing description, and that is therefore exemplified by all of the internal state-tokens for which "olfactory sensation" stands. After we have made this determination, we are able to check to see whether "olfactory sensation" can be ascribed to an internal state-token without investigating the causal history of the token. We need only check to see whether it is an instance of α.

13 A closely related view, which I regard as only marginally inferior to the view recommended here, is that "olfactory sensation" is synonymous with "sensation of the type ψ such that (1) ψ is nomologically connected with types of stimuli that act on odor-detecting sense organs, and (2) ψ is not nomologically connected with types of stimuli that act on sense organs of other kinds." (The difference between the two views is just that the second one has the quasifunctional term "odor-detecting sense organ" in place of the anatomical term "nose." I prefer the first view to the second one for reasons of uniformity. When one turns from "olfactory sensation" to "visual sensation," one has a hard time finding an appropriate counterpart of the second suggestion.)

There is an objection to the second view that should be answered. This objection is based on the perception that the content of the term "odor" derives at least in part from the content of "olfactory sensation"; that either "odor" is introduced as a synonym for expressions like "power of producing olfactory sensations," or we use an expression like this one in fixing the reference of "odor." Of course, if this perception were correct, it could not be the case that "olfactory sensation" is synonymous with an expression that contains "odor." However, I question the validity of the perception. Even if it is true that we have to invoke olfactory sensory states in some way in conferring content on "odor," it by no means follows that we have to use the term "olfactory sensation" in invoking them. An alternative suggestion, which I find more plausible, is that we invoke them by mobilizing one or more of the infralinguistic concepts that stand for types of olfactory sensations. Moreover, it is not obvious that we have to invoke olfactory sensations in conferring content on "odor." Perhaps it is enough to learn to use this term under the influence of olfactory sensations, where "using under the influence of ψ's" differs from "invoking ψ's" in that it refers to a subpersonal and largely mechanical process that does not require one to mobilize a term or a concept that stands for ψ's.

184

Although it is clear that we can recognize instances of α by introspection, it is not entirely clear how we do so. Do we use an infralinguistic concept that stands for α or do we use a variety of infralinguistic concepts that stand for more tightly circumscribed characteristics? It isn't obvious how this question should be answered. Unlike the qualitative characteristics that guide our application of "sensation of heat" and other basic descriptions, α is not a universal of the standard sort: It is not the case that all instances of α can be said to resemble each other. (Compare the sensation you get when you encounter the smell of frying bacon with the sensation produced by the aroma of honeysuckle.) All that can be said is that every two instances of α are linked by the ancestral of a phenomenal similarity relation.[14] Thus, α is in a sense halfway between a characteristic like *being a pain* and a characteristic like *being a sensation*. It is more like *being a pain* than like *being a sensation* in that its instances are connected by a phenomenal similarity relation, but it is different than *being a pain* in that its instances are not *directly* linked by the relation in question. Do we have infralinguistic concepts that stand for state-types of this sort? It is not entirely clear.

Fortunately, our purpose here does not require us to reach a conclusion about this issue. Even if we do not have a qualitative concept that stands for α itself, it is clear that we have qualitative concepts for a number of more narrowly circumscribed types of olfactory sensations. These concepts provide an adequate basis for explaining how we are able to determine by introspection alone whether "olfactory sensation" is ascribable to an internal state-token. (Recall that we were able to explain introspection-based ascriptions of "sensation" without postulating a qualitative concept that stands for *being a sensation*.)

14 Where π is a phenomenal similarity relation, the ancestral of π is a relation λ that meets this condition: A sensation x bears λ to a sensation y if and only if it is possible for there to be a finite series of sensations such that x and y are the two end points of the series and every intermediate member of the series bears the relation π to the sensations that are adjacent to it.

8

Concepts of visual sensations:
Their content and their deployment

This chapter is concerned with questions about the forms and limits of our cognitive access to visual sensations, and with questions about the semantic properties of the concepts on which such access depends.

It is convenient to distinguish at the outset between two types of visual sensations. First, there are sensations that have the power to induce us to form perceptual beliefs about the visually perceptible properties of extramental objects and events. The members of this group, which will hereafter be called *belief-generating sensations*, include all of the sensations that occur in the course of everyday veridical visual perception. But the group has other members as well. Specifically, because we can be led to form perceptual beliefs – or, if you prefer, quasiperceptual beliefs – when we are dreaming and also when we are hallucinating, the group includes sensations that are involved in dreams and hallucinations. Second, there are visual sensations that lack the power to induce us to form perceptual beliefs. These sensations include after-images of various kinds and also the highly amorphous visual sensations that come to the fore when we close our eyes. I will refer to members of this second group as *perceptually barren* sensations.

In defining belief-generating sensations I said that they are sensations that have the *power* to generate perceptual beliefs. I defined them in this way because I want it to be possible for a visual sensation to count as a belief-generating sensation even if it doesn't actually bring a perceptual belief into existence. But what is meant by "power to cause perceptual beliefs"? Here is a definition: A visual sensation has the power to cause perceptual beliefs if it exemplifies some type ϕ such that sensations of type ϕ normally cause perceptual beliefs unless their owners happen not to be paying attention to the visible portion of the

I thank Sydney Shoemaker and Lynn Stephens for a number of illuminating conversations about the topics discussed in this chapter.

world, or their owners happen to have special reasons for doubting that things are as they appear.

Apart from a few paragraphs at the end of the chapter, I will focus on belief-generating sensations. Barren sensations present a number of problems that are eminently deserving of careful attention, but I will not discuss these problems here.

There are two groups of questions that I will discuss. First, what is the nature of our awareness of belief-generating sensations? Can it appropriately be described as *direct*? (That is to say, can it be maintained that our awareness of belief-generating sensations is fully immediate in the sense in which our awareness of pain is fully immediate?) Second, what is the nature of the concepts we use in characterizing our belief-generating sensations? What are their semantic properties?

(An aside: Although I have just promised a discussion of semantic issues, the reader will find that I have comparatively little to say that bears directly on questions about content. Most of the paragraphs in this chapter are concerned with questions about awareness. But actually it is necessary to discuss these questions in order to keep my promise. This is because the most important semantic question about our concepts of visual sensations is the question of whether any of these concepts are like the concept of pain in being infratheoretical. My answer to this question is negative; and, as it turns out, it is impossible to justify this answer without taking a long look at certain questions about awareness (and in particular, at the question of whether awareness of belief-generating sensations is direct or inferential).)

I will be exclusively concerned with visual sensations. However, I believe that much of what I will say is applicable, mutatis mutandis, to auditory sensations as well.

I

The first thesis I wish to recommend is the proposition that awareness of belief-generating sensations does not normally play a role in visual perception. Belief-generating sensations are *diaphanous* – they mediate our awareness of extramental objects and extramental states of affairs, but normally they are not objects of awareness in their own right. Normally, for example, when one is seeing a barn, it does not cross one's mind that one has visual sensations that count as representations of the barn.

This thesis is widely esteemed. It is, for example, defended at some length in a recent paper by Gilbert Harman. Harman focuses on a case in which a certain subject, Eloise, is looking at a tree. He writes:

> In the case of a painting Eloise can be aware of those features of the painting that are responsible for its being a painting of a unicorn. That is, she can turn her attention to the pattern of a paint on the canvas by virtue of which the painting represents a unicorn. But in the case of her visual experience of a tree, I want to say that she is not aware of, as it were, the mental paint by virtue of which her experience is an experience of seeing a tree. . . .
>
> Some sense datum theorists will object that Eloise is indeed aware of the relevant mental paint when she is aware of an arrangement of color, because these sense datum theorists assert that the color she is aware of is inner and mental and not a property of external objects. But, this sense datum claim is counter to ordinary visual experience. When Eloise sees a tree before her, the colors she experiences are all experienced as features of the tree and its surroundings. None of them are experienced as intrinsic features of her experience. Nor does she experience any features of anything as intrinsic features of her experience. And that is true of you too. There is nothing special about Eloise's visual experience. When you see a tree, you do not experience any features as intrinsic features of your experience. Look at a tree and try to turn your attention to intrinsic features of your visual experience. I predict you will find that the only features there to turn your attention to will be features of the presented tree. . . .[1]

Harman goes on to make similar claims about other forms of sense experience. He maintains that we are not aware of the intrinsic features of any of our sensations. I think that this is wrong. However, I endorse everything that he says in the admirably clear and persuasive passage I have just quoted.

In denying that we are directly aware of belief-generating sensations when we visually perceive something, I am taking a side in the debate between advocates of the so-called *representational* theory of perception and defenders of the theory that is known as *direct realism*. According to representationalism, perception of extramental states of affairs involves two forms of awareness, one direct and the other indirect. When one perceives a barn, one is directly aware of a visual sensation that counts as a representation of the barn, and one is indirectly aware of the barn itself. Further, one is indirectly aware of the barn by virtue of being

1 Gilbert Harman, "The Intrinsic Quality of Experience," read at the 1987 Chapel Hill Colloquium in Philosophy, October 17, 1987.

directly aware of the sensation. On the other hand, direct realism maintains that perception involves just one form of awareness. A direct realist will normally grant that we have sensations when we perceive the extramental world, and that it is in some sense true that we perceive the extramental world in virtue of having sensations. But a direct realist will deny that perception involves awareness of sensations. According to a direct realist, when one perceives a barn one is directly aware of the barn.

When it is taken as a thesis about perception by touch, taste, or smell, representationalism is largely correct. Often we do not bother to focus on our sensations when we are attending to an extramental state of affairs by one of these forms of perception, but we can generally be said to be at least marginally aware of them. Further, there are times when this awareness is extremely vivid. For example, when I am aware of a peanut butter cookie I am more aware of the taste sensation than of the partially masticated cookie in my mouth.

But representationalism does not claim only that we are aware of sensations in addition to being aware of extramental objects: it maintains that we are aware of the latter by virtue of being aware of the former. What about this claim? Is it correct when taken as a thesis about tactual awareness? And when taken as a thesis about gustatory awareness? And when taken as a thesis about olfactory awareness? Although I cannot defend this position here, I hold that the answer is affirmative in all three cases. To be sure, one does not often consciously infer the existence of an extramental particular from the existence of a sensation. Typically, one does not think "Aha! Here is a tactual (gustatory, olfactory) sensation of type ϕ, so I must be touching (tasting, smelling) something of type ψ." However, as I see it, when one is concerned to *justify* a belief to the effect that one is perceiving an extramental entity by touch (taste, smell), it is necessary to cite one or more of one's tactual (gustatory, olfactory) sensations in giving the justification.

As far as I can tell, however, even if representationalism gives us a more or less correct account of tactual, gustatory, and olfactory awareness, it is completely wrong when taken as a view about visual and auditory perception. For adequate accounts of these two forms of perception we must look to the writings of the direct realists.

So much for my first thesis – the claim that we do not normally apprehend visual sensations when we are visually perceiving the environment. To state my second thesis I need a technical term. Let us agree

to say that *x* is *entertaining a visual appearance* if it is true either (1) that
there is something that looks ϕ to *x*, where ϕ is a visually accessible
property such as *being blue* or *being square*, or (2) that it looks to *x* as if *p*,
where *p* is a proposition that ascribes some visually accessible property
to a visually manifest particular. Using this notion, my second thesis
can be expressed as follows: We do not normally apprehend visual
sensations in the course of entertaining appearances. I have no wish to
deny that we *have* visual sensations in the course of entertaining appearances; indeed it seems clear that entertaining an appearance consists in
having a visual sensation. Rather the point is that we are not *aware of*
visual sensations when we entertain appearances. To be aware of a
sensation one must register its existence at the level of belief; and it is
certain that entertainings of visual appearances are not normally accompanied by beliefs about visual sensations.

There is a sense in which this second thesis is largely contained in my
first thesis. Thus, it is impossible to perceive something visually without entertaining a visual appearance: When it is true that someone is
perceiving something, it is inevitably true as well that there is something that appears in a certain way to the individual in question. Now
my first thesis asserts that we are not normally aware of visual sensations when we are visually perceiving the environment. Thus, if the
first thesis is true, there is a class of cases in which we are entertaining
visual appearances but in which we are not aware of visual sensations –
specifically, the cases in which entertainings of visual appearances are
associated with perceptual states. But now, my second thesis claims
that it is true in general – that is, in all normal cases – that we are not
aware of visual sensations when we are entertaining visual appearances.
It follows that much of the content of my second thesis is contained
implicitly in my first thesis. However, the second thesis is not entirely
redundant, for there are cases in which we entertain visual appearances
but in which the entertainings cannot be said to be associated with
perceptual states. Thus, for example, even though an object looks blue
to me, I may still fail to judge that it is blue. In a case of this sort I am
entertaining an appearance but I cannot be said to perceive that an
object is blue.

My third thesis, which is closely related to the second, is a claim
about the psychological state one is in when one believes that one is
entertaining a visual appearance. Specifically, it is the claim that such
beliefs are not normally accompanied by apprehensions of visual sensations. To believe that one is entertaining an appearance is to believe

either that something looks ϕ to one, where ϕ is as before, or to believe that it looks to one as if p, where p is as before. Normally, when one has a belief of either of these forms, it does not cross one's mind that one is having a visual sensation. To be sure, one does have a sensation, and the sensation plays a role in causing one's belief, but one takes no note of the sensation. The sensation lives and dies without recognition.

To summarize: According to my first three theses, we are not normally aware of visual sensations when we see things, nor when we entertain visual appearances, nor when we believe that we are entertaining appearances. On the other hand, following in the footsteps of many others, I have maintained that we have visual sensations when we see things, and also when we entertain appearances, and also when we believe that we are entertaining appearances.

Now in view of my three negative theses about awareness of visual sensations, it is appropriate to ask for a justification for my positive claims about the existence of visual sensations. After all, if we are not directly aware of visual sensations, there is logical room for skepticism about their existence. My reply to this worry is as follows: We are justified in believing in visual sensations of which we are not directly aware because we are justified in believing in folk psychology. Folk psychology contains laws that link the notion of a visual appearance to the notion of a visual sensation. To be more specific, it contains laws that can be formulated roughly as follows:

> If it looks to x as if p, then x is having a sensation of the sort that x would be having if the conditions of observation were standard and x was seeing that p. (1)

> If y looks to x the way ϕ-things look when x sees them under standard conditions of observation, then x is having a sensation of the sort that x has when x sees a ϕ-thing under standard conditions of observation. (2)

> If y looks to x the way ϕ-things look when normal observers see them under standard conditions of observation, then x is having a sensation of the sort that normal observers have when they see ϕ-things under standard conditions of observation. (3)

Because of these laws, if we are justified in believing in folk psychology, we are also justified in believing that visual sensations are involved in our entertainings of visual appearances. But it is clear that we are justified in believing in folk psychology, for it has served us well on countless occasions.

Now if the foregoing theses are correct, then in the normal course of things we are not aware of our belief-generating sensations. This can be put another way by saying that awareness of belief-generating sensations is not something that arises spontaneously, but only as a result of special prompting. The forms that the special prompting may take are various – one may, for example, be led to think of one's belief-generating sensations by theoretical concerns, such as the concerns that are occupying our attention in this chapter, or by a line of thought that is triggered by a visit to one's ophthalmologist. But special prompting of some sort is required.

This brings us to my fourth thesis, which is a claim about the psychological processes by which beliefs about belief-generating sensations are brought into existence. In my case, I find, what happens is this: As a result of special prompting, I consciously ask myself a question like "What sort of visual sensations am I having now?" or "Am I having a visual sensation of type ϕ?" I then take note of how things look to me; I take stock of my current entertainings of visual appearances. Having canvassed my current entertainings, and having formed an adequate set of beliefs about them, I obtain an answer to my question by inferring a proposition about my current sensory state from these beliefs. Thus, for example, if I find that something currently looks blue to me, I infer that I am currently having a sensation of the sort that I normally have when I see a blue object. Or I infer a closely related proposition, such as the proposition that I am having a sensation *of* blue.

Now in drawing conclusions of these sorts, I am not consciously aware of basing my inferences on any beliefs other than beliefs about my current entertainings of appearances. But beliefs about my current entertainings are not sufficient grounds for conclusions about sensations. Hence, as they present themselves to my consciousness, the inferences in question are fallacious. However, there is a sense in which the inferences are entirely legitimate. In addition to my conscious beliefs about my current entertainings, I also have tacit beliefs that link the notion of a visual appearance to the notion of a visual sensation. Thus, among other tacit beliefs of this sort, I have tacit beliefs that can be expressed by (1)–(3). When they are combined with my conscious beliefs about my current entertainings of appearances, these tacit beliefs provide deductively adequate justifications for conclusions about my visual sensations. I have no idea whether the tacit beliefs in question should be thought of as playing a causal role in the formation of such beliefs; for there is no reason to think that the processes that underlie belief-formation must always follow the paths that are commended to our attention by the canons of deductive logic. However, the existence of these tacit beliefs makes it appropriate for me to draw conclusions about my sensations from my beliefs about entertainings of appearances. Because of the tacit beliefs, even though I cannot be said to be consciously aware of full justifications for my conclusions about my sensations, I can be said to be in possession of full justifications.

If this account of the process of becoming aware of one's belief-generating sensations is correct, there is a significant difference between awareness of bodily sensations such as pain and awareness of visual sensations. Awareness of pain is direct, and awareness of visual sensations is inferential.

Let us turn now to my fifth thesis, which postulates a second significant difference. As we saw in the previous chapter, we have concepts of bodily sensations that are infratheoretical. However, according to my fifth thesis, just the opposite is true in the case of belief-generating sensations. The concepts we use to apprehend belief-generating sensations are higly theoretical, in the sense that they presuppose the truth of folk psychology. Thus, in my case at least, the concepts that are involved in awareness of belief-generating sensations are always of the same type as the concepts expressed by "sensation of red," "sensation of the sort I normally have when I see a red object," and "sensation of the sort that normal observers have when they see objects that are red." Hence, such concepts always have the notion of a sensation as a constituent. Now, as we observed in the previous chapter, the notion of a sensation is one that presupposes the truth of folk psychology. Moreover, it is evident that if one concept has a second concept as a constituent, and the second concept presupposes the truth of a theory, the first concept presupposes the truth of the theory as well. It follows that the concepts expressed by "sensation of red," and so on are theoretical.

There is also a second reason for thinking that the concepts in question are theoretical. Thus, consider the concept expressed by "sensation of red." Evidently, it has a constituent corresponding to the phrase "of red." It is not entirely clear what should be said about the semantic properties of this phrase. I favor the view that it is coextensive with "of a sort that a normal human observer has when he or she sees a red object under standard conditions of perception." However the details do not matter here. It is clear that we must embrace some form of the view that "of red" classifies sensations in terms of a nonphenomenological relation to an extramental property, the property *being a case of red*. (By a nonphenomenological relation I mean one that cannot be seen to obtain by direct awareness – one that can only be apprehended by the lens provided by a theory.)

It is clear, I think, that the same is true of the phrases "of the sort I normally have when I see a red object" and "of the sort that normal observers have when they see objects that are red." Like "of red," each of these descriptions classifies sensations in terms of a nonphenomenological relation to an extramental property.

II

My first three theses can be summarized by saying that in the normal course of things we are not aware of our belief-generating sensations. This proposition is in no sense new; together with other propositions of the same ilk, it has been much discussed in the debates between direct realists and advocates of representationalism.

Now in the course of these debates the advocates of representationalism have raised a number of objections to the proposition, and some of these objections can be quite persuasive. In this section I will discuss the four objections that have seemed to me at one time or another to have the greatest chance of success.

First objection. When one is dreaming or one is subject to an hallucination, one is certainly aware of *something*. However, one is not aware of extramental particulars of any kind. Hence, one must be aware of certain of one's sensations. Moreover, what one is aware of in such cases is similar in kind to what one is aware of in cases of veridical perception. Hence, it must be true that in cases of veridical perception one is aware of sensations.

Further, it would be counterintuitive to say that one is *only* aware of sensations in cases of the second kind. Hence, it is necessary to distinguish between two forms of visual awareness, direct and indirect. In describing a case of veridical visual perception, we should say that a subject is directly aware of a visual sensation and indirectly aware of an extramental object or event.

Reply. I reject the first premise. I grant, of course, that it seems that one is aware of something when one is dreaming. Equally, I grant that it seems that one is aware of something when one is hallucinating. But these appearances are misleading.

To be aware of a sensation it is necessary to be aware *that* some proposition concerning the sensation is true. Hence, if one is aware of a sensation in the course of a dream, it must be the case that one is subsuming the sensation under one or more concepts that stand for types of sensations. But in normal cases of dreaming one is doing nothing of the kind. In normal cases, sensations are the farthest things from one's mind. In dreaming, one does not make use of concepts that stand for types of sensation, but rather of concepts that stand for extramental entities of various kinds. And the same is true in cases in which one is hallucinating – or at least, it is true in such cases until one comes to realize that a hallucination is in progress. After Macbeth comes to understand that there is no dagger in front of him, he has a reason to form the belief that he is experiencing a visual sensation of a dagger. And after he forms this belief, he can be said to be aware of something. But prior to the moment of forming the belief, he is not aware of anything – however much it may seem to him otherwise. For, prior to that moment, he has not activated any concepts that stand for sensations. Prior to that moment, his attention is directed outward. The only concepts he is using are concepts that stand for extramental entities.

Second objection. When one is aware of two extramental objects that exemplify the same color, one is aware of a resemblance. Either one is aware of a fact involving the objects themselves and a physical similarity relation, or one is aware of a fact involving the sensations that represent the objects and a phenomenal similarity relation. However, a careful inventory of the possible candidates shows that there is no physical similarity relation with the right properties. It is just not true that any two extramental particulars that exemplify the same color will be found to resemble one another by virtue of their physical characteristics. Hence, contrary to what direct realism maintains, it must be the case that our awareness of extramental objects depends on awareness of sensations. When it seems to one that one is directly aware of a fact involving two colored physical objects and a physical similarity relation, one is making a mistake. It is true that one is aware of physical objects, but one's awareness of them is only indirect. One's awareness of them derives from awareness of the sensations that represent them. Moreover, the only similarity relation of which one is aware is a relation that links these sensations. In taking this relation to be physical one is projecting an internal fact onto the external world.[2]

Because it denies that physical objects that exemplify the same color are always similar in physical properties, this argument runs counter to common sense. However, it appears that the denial is strongly supported by empirical facts. A robin's egg, the sky, a band of a rainbow, and the surface of a lake are all blue, but there is no physical universal that is common to all of them. Nor is it true that all objects that exemplify the same color reflect light with the same wavelength: "Objects with identical [reflection] spectra will, to be sure, look to be the same color, but indefinitely large numbers of objects that are spectrally different will also look to be the same color; it is unlikely that any two things chosen at random which look to have the same blue color under normal conditions will have identical reflection spectra. . . ."[3]

Reply. The first premise of this argument stacks the deck by describing the facts in a way that is maximally favorable to representationalism. Suppose you see two objects that are both blue. According to the point of view that is represented by the first premise, you should describe this situation by saying that you are aware of a fact involving a similarity relation. But there is also a more neutral way of describing the situation: You can say instead that the objects *look* similar. To be sure, it is necessary to appeal to a similarity relation in explaining why the objects look similar to you. It is necessary to say that they look similar by virtue of the fact that they are represented by sensations that are similar. But it is possible to explain the apparent similarity of the objects in terms of the similarity of the sensations without claiming that the similarity of the sensations is an object of awareness. The apparent similarity of the objects can be explained by saying that their looking similar consists in the fact that they are represented by similar sensations.

But wait! Doesn't this defense concede too much? Suppose it is true that looking similar consists in being represented by similar sensations. Doesn't it follow that when one is aware that two objects look similar one is aware that they are represented by similar sensations? If so, the defense is worthless. For it implicitly concedes the main point at issue.

2 Versions of this argument can be found in a number of places. See, for example, Moreland Perkins, *Sensing the World* (Indianapolis: Hackett Publishing Company, 1983), pp. 235–39.
3 Clyde L. Hardin, *Color for Philosophers* (Indianapolis: Hackett Publishing Company, 1988), p. 7.

This worry presupposes a general principle that can easily be seen to be false. The principle I have in mind can be formulated as follows: If the truth of p consists in the truth of q, then, provided one is in possession of the concepts involved in the proposition that q as well as the concepts involved in the proposition that p, when one is aware that p is true, one must be aware that q is true. The problem with this principle is that one may be in full possession of the concepts involved in the proposition that q without being disposed to deploy them on the same occasions on which one deploys the concepts involved in the proposition that p. Consider, for example, someone who is in full possession of the concept of H_2O but who is not disposed to make use of this concept when spotting a glass of water. That person will always be aware of glasses of water as glasses of water – never as glasses of H_2O.

Third objection. Suppose that *McX*'s visual sensation-types exchange their representational properties, with the result that, for example, the *McX*ian sensation-type that used to represent yellow now comes to represent blue. Suppose also that the nonrepresentational properties of *McX*'s sensation-types are not affected by the change. Thus, for example, the state-type that used to represent blue retains its power to activate *McX*'s visual memories of the blue things he has seen in the past. Because of this second assumption, it seems reasonable to think that *McX* will be able to determine from the inside that objects no longer have the same effects on him as they used to have. He will be able to tell from the inside that a spectrum inversion has occurred. But this means that he will be aware of the intrinsic natures of his sensations.

Reply. *McX* can determine that a spectrum inversion has occurred without taking note of his sensations. He need only take note of the appearances of things. For example, he can determine that an inversion has occurred by observing that the things that used to look blue now look yellow.

Fourth objection. In *Sense and Content*, Christopher Peacocke argues that there are forms of everyday awareness that have to be seen as awareness of features of belief-generating sensations.[4] That is to say, he maintains that there are aspects of our everyday visual experience such that (1) we can be said to be directly aware of these aspects, and (2) our awareness of them depends essentially on the deployment of sensory concepts. In defense of (2), he urges that it is impossible to express our

4 Christopher Peacocke, *Sense and Content* (Oxford: Oxford University Press, 1983).

awareness of the aspects in question using only the language of appearances (that is, using terms like "looks" and "appears" in preference to terms that stand for types of sensation). He writes:

> Suppose you are standing on a road which stretches from you in a straight line to the horizon. There are two trees at the roadside, one a hundred yards from you, the other two hundred. Your experience represents these objects as being of the same physical height and other dimensions; that is, taking your experience at face value you would judge that the trees are roughly the same physical size. . . . Yet there is also some sense in which the nearer tree occupies more of your visual field than the more distant tree. This is as much a feature of your experience as is its representing the trees as being the same height.[5]

In this case, Peacocke is saying, there is a difference that can be called a difference in size. However, it is not a difference in physical size, for it is stipulated that the physical sizes of the two trees are the same. Nor is it a difference in apparent size: If one were concerned to describe the appearances of the two trees, one would have to say that they look to be the same size. So we have to explain the difference in size by appealing to the intrinsic qualities of the sensations that represent the trees. We have to say that one of these sensations fills a larger portion of the visual field than the other.

If all of this is true, and it is also true that we can be directly aware of differences like this difference in size, then it must be true that we can be directly aware of our visual sensations.

Reply. The language of appearances is a much more complicated and flexible instrument than the objection allows. Although it is true that the two trees look to be the same size, this does not preclude our using the language of appearances to capture the difference in size to which Peacocke calls our attention.

Let us start by considering a simpler case. When we perceive people on the ground from the top of a tall building, we may say that they look like ants. But we may also say that they look much larger than ants – that they look like people of normal size. These two claims are compatible because "look" has a different sense in the first claim than it does in the second. The first claim is a short form of the proposition that the people on the ground look the way ants look when they are seen from small distances. The second claim is a short form of the proposition that

---

5 Peacocke, ibid., p. 12.

198

the people on the ground look much larger than ants look when ants are seen from a great distance. Thus, "looks" is governed by a tacit adverbial qualifier in each of the claims, and the claims are compatible because the tacit adverbial qualifier that governs it in the first claim is different than the one that governs it in the second claim.

It is much the same in the case that Peacocke cites. It is possible to say that Peacocke's two trees look to be the same size and also that the first tree looks larger than the second. These statements are compatible because "looks" invokes a different adverbial qualifier in the first statement than it does in the second. When we say that the two trees look to be the same size, we mean that they look the way trees that are the same size look when they are seen from different distances. And when we say that the first tree looks larger than the second, we mean that the first tree looks roughly the way that a tree that is larger than the second tree would look if it were the same distance from the observer as the second tree. It is clear that there is no incompatibility here. Accordingly, it seems that we can use the language of appearances to express all of the relevant facts about comparative size.

It seems to me that the language of appearances is the source of our most fundamental characterizations of Peacockean phenomena. It is true that we can also characterize such phenomena by speaking of facts involving visual sensations, but it seems to me that we arrive at such characterizations by inference. Having observed, for example, that the people on the ground look like ants, one may go on to affirm that the sensations by which the people are represented occupy comparatively small areas of the visual field. As I see it, this proposition about the visual field can only be obtained by inference. It would be a mistake to think that it is shown to be true by the data of immediate awareness.

III

I put forward five theses in section I about awareness of belief-generating sensations and the content of the concepts that are involved in such awareness. As I mentioned in the previous section, the first three of these theses can be summarized by the proposition that in the normal course of things we are not aware of belief-generating sensations. The fourth thesis is the claim that we become aware of belief-generating sensations by inferring propositions about them from our beliefs about entertainings of visual appearances. And the fifth thesis is the claim that the content of our concepts of belief-generating sensations is highly theoretical, in the sense that it derives from the relationship that these concepts bear to the laws of folk psychology.

Although, when taken together, these theses may be said to provide an account of the nature of awareness of belief-generating sensations, this account is extremely sketchy. In this section I will supplement the account by adding two new theses. These additional theses seem to me to be inherently plausible, but neither of them can be said to be so plausible that it does not require a defense. Unfortunately, it would take us too far afield to consider supporting arguments here. Thus, relative to this work, these additional theses have the status of speculations.

In order to state my first speculation, I need the notion of a *visual belief*. Where B is a belief, let us say that the content of B is visual if (1) B attributes one or more visually accessible properties and/or relations to one or more visually manifest particulars, or (2) B is a belief to the effect that one is seeing one or more visually manifest particulars, or (3) B is a belief to the effect that one is seeing that p, where p is a proposition that attributes one or more visually accessible properties and/or relations to one or more particulars, or (4) B is a belief to the effect that one is entertaining an appearance. Further, let us say that B is a visual belief if its content is visual and it is caused by visual inputs in the way that beliefs with visual content are standardly caused.

The first speculation is a hypothesis about what it is that justifies visual beliefs. According to this speculation, when we say that a visual belief is justified, we are asserting that it is justified – in part, at least – by an appearance that the believer is currently entertaining. More concretely, according to the first speculation, if one were to say that one of the following visual beliefs is justified:

> Vola's belief that the object in front of her is blue
>
> Vola's belief that she is seeing a blue object
>
> Vola's belief that she sees that the object in front of her is blue
>
> Vola's belief that the object in front of her looks blue

one would be claiming that there is something that currently looks blue to Vola, and that its looking blue to her provides her with at least part of the justification for her belief.

Actually, what I have just said is only an approximation to the doctrine I wish to recommend. Strictly speaking, the doctrine is not the claim that one's visual beliefs are justified by facts that consist of objects' appearing in some way to one, but is rather the claim that the beliefs are justified by what might be called the subjective components of such facts. When a certain object looks blue to a subject, the subject is in a psychological state that can also occur when it is not the case that something is looking blue to him or to her. Thus, the subject is also in the state in question when he or she is dreaming that there is something blue in front of him or her, and also when he or she is having an hallucination to the same effect. The state in question is the state that is common to all those cases in which it looks to the subject as if there is something blue in front of him or her. So as to have a name for this state, let us follow Chisholm in calling it the *state of being appeared blue to*.[6] Further, let us agree to say that the state of being appeared blue to and all other states of the same sort are *look-sustaining* states.

Putting this new terminology to use, I can express my first speculation as follows: If a visual belief is justified, its justification consists – in part, at least – in the fact that the believer is in a look-sustaining state of the appropriate sort. For example, according to the first speculation, if Vola is justified in holding one of the beliefs cited two paragraphs ago, it must be true that Vola is in the state of being looked blue to. Further, her justification for the belief must consist – in part, at least – in the fact that she is in this state.

Look-sustaining states are sensory states. They are not doxastic states, nor do they have doxastic states as components. Accordingly, the first speculation implies that if a visual belief is justified, its justification derives – in part, at least – from a state that is not a belief.

6 See, for example: Roderick M. Chisholm, *Perceiving* (Ithaca: Cornell University Press, 1957), pp. 61–64; and Chisholm, *Theory of Knowledge*, 2nd ed. (Englewood Cliffs, NJ: Prentice Hall, 1977), pp. 26–30. As readers of Chisholm will have recognized, my debt to him involves much more than terminology. The view that I am calling "my first speculation" has long been championed by Chisholm. (It is defended with considerable subtlety in the works I have just cited. See also Roderick M. Chisholm, *The Foundations of Knowing* (Minneapolis: The University of Minnesota Press, 1982), pp. 134–45.)

Incidentally, in stating the first speculation, I mean to be using "looks" in what Chisholm sometimes calls its "phenomenological" sense. See Chisholm, *Theory of Knowledge*, p. 27. For more on the various senses of "looks," see Frank Jackson, *Perception* (Cambridge: Cambridge University Press, 1977), Chapter 2. (Jackson's term "phenomenal sense" is evidently equivalent to Chisholm's term "phenomenological sense.")

Thus, the first speculation commits us to a picture of justification that might be called nondoxastic foundationalism.[7]

This brings us to the second speculation, which is a thesis about the ultimate metaphysical nature of look-sustaining states. According to this view, where S is any subject, the fact consisting of S's being in a look-sustaining state is identical with a fact that consists, first, in S's having one or more visual sensations, and second, in these sensations exemplifying one or more qualitative characteristics and/or relations. Thus, for example, the view claims that the fact consisting of S's being appeared blue to is the fact that consists of S's having one or more visual sensations that exemplify the property *being a case of phenomenal blue* (that is, the intrinsic property of sensations that is nomologically connected, in normal subjects, with seeing blue objects under the conditions of observation that count as standard in the actual world). This view can also be expressed by saying that look-sustaining states can be apprehended under two quite different kinds of description. Thus, the view can be seen as claiming that, although we originally apprehend look-sustaining states under descriptions that are couched in terms of the language of appearing, they can also be apprehended under descriptions that represent them as facts involving sensations.[8-10]

7 Nondoxastic foundationalism is closely related to a view that John Pollock defends (under the name *nondoxastic internalism*) in *Contemporary Theories of Knowledge* (Totowa, NJ: Rowman and Littlefield, 1986). Pollock writes as follows (p. 91):

> Externalist theories depart radically from traditional doxastic theories. . . . Nondoxastic internalist theories, however, may be structures very similar to classical foundations theories. For instance, *direct realism* is the view that perceptual states can license perceptual judgments about physical objects directly and without mediation by beliefs about the perceptual states. Direct realism can have a structure very much like a foundations theory. My own view is that the foundations theory sketched in chapter two gets things almost right. Where it goes wrong is in adopting the doxastic assumption and thereby assuming that perceptual input must be mediated by epistemologically basic beliefs. It now seems clear that epistemic norms can appeal directly to our being in perceptual states and need not appeal to our having beliefs to that effect.

8 Note that to defend this second speculation it would be necessary to do more than appeal to (1)–(3).

9 If it is true that S's being in a look-sustaining state is identical with S's having a sensation of a certain sort, why isn't S aware of a sensation when S is in a look-sustaining state? Why isn't S aware of the state as a state that involves one or more sensations? It seems likely that the answer has something to do with the fact that the qualitative characteristics of visual sensations are such as to create the impression of three-dimensionality. But I cannot develop this suggestion here. (There are, however, a few observations about the three-dimensionality of visual sensations at the end of section V.)

When these two speculations are combined with the theses that were presented in section I, we obtain an account of the justification of beliefs about belief-generating sensations that runs as follows. Suppose that a subject, S, holds a well-justified belief, B_1, to the effect that S is currently having a sensation of blue. Suppose also that B_1 is true. By the fourth of the five theses presented earlier, this belief is inferred from a second belief, B_2, to the effect that something now looks blue to S (or from some related belief, such as the belief that it now looks to S as if something in front of S is blue). It follows that part of S's justification for B_1 derives from B_2. (Not all of S's justification for B_1 derives from B_2. As we saw in section I, when a belief like B_1 is inferred from a belief like B_2, part of the justification for the former belief comes from laws of folk psychology (such as (1)–(3) earlier) that link the notion of an appearance to the notion of a visual sensation. Here, however, I will ignore the folk psychological component of S's justification for B_1.) Now, by hypothesis, B_1 is fully justified. Accordingly, because its justification derives in part from B_2, B_2 must be fully justified. But according to our first speculation, if a belief like B_2 is justified, its justification must derive – in part, at least – from a look-sustaining state of the believer. Hence, we may be sure that S is now being appeared blue to, and that this fact provides part of S's justification for B_2. But because S's justification for B_1 derives from B_2, we may also be sure that S's justification for B_1 derives in part from the fact that S is now being appeared blue to. Further, by the second speculation, the fact that S is being appeared blue to is, unbeknown to S, identical with the fact that S currently has a visual sensation with a certain intrinsic nature. It follows that unbeknown to S, S's justification for B_1 derives in part from the fact that S currently has a sensation with the intrinsic nature in question. Moreover, this sensation is exactly the one that makes B_1 true. So we can draw this final conclusion: Part of S's

---

10 It seems that there is a use of "aware of" such that if S is aware that p, and p is identical with the fact that q, then S may be said to be aware of the fact that q – even if it would be wrong to say that S is aware that q. If there is such a use, then, provided that the second speculation is correct, it is possible to say, truly, that one is aware of a fact involving one or more visual sensations when one is aware that one is entertaining a visual appearance. However, it should be clear that this has no tendency to undermine the conclusions reached in sections I and II.

justification for B_1 derives from the existence and the intrinsic nature of the very sensation that makes B_1 true.

The reader will recognize in this conclusion a pattern that we discerned in Chapter 5. As we noticed there, it is a characteristic feature of introspective beliefs about pains (and of introspective beliefs about all of the other sensations to which we have direct access) that they receive their justification from sensations that are identical with the sensations that make them true. Our current finding can be expressed by saying that, if the two speculations are correct, then this same generalization holds – albeit with qualifications – for introspective beliefs that are concerned with sensations to which we do not have direct access.

IV

We have found reason to accept the proposition that there are sensations of which we are not directly aware, for we have found reason to believe that belief-generating sensations lie outside the realm of direct awareness. By the same token, we have found reason to reject the familiar idea that accessibility to direct awareness can serve as a criterion of the sensory. This quasi-Cartesian criterion is much too restrictive.

Another conclusion we can draw is that it is necessary to separate the notions of introspection and direct awareness – even with respect to sensations. We have found no reason to deny that there is introspective access to belief-generating sensations; on the contrary, we have noticed that there is a plausible – if somewhat speculative – account of awareness of belief-generating sensations that implies that such awareness more or less fits the account of introspective awareness that is given in Chapter 5. Thus, our findings about direct awareness show that the introspectible realm is much broader in extent than the realm of direct awareness.

Finally, we can conclude that some of the most important traditional epistemologies have been on the wrong track. Cartesian philosophy presupposes that it is possible to be directly aware of one's belief-generating sensations, and the same is true of several varieties of classical empiricism. It is also true of several varieties of phenomenalism. It appears that these theories must be rejected – not on conceptual grounds, but because they misrepresent the nature of visual perception.

204

Before bringing this chapter to a close, I will say a few words about the relationship between belief-generating sensations and barren sensations. (The notion of a barren sensation is introduced on the first page of this chapter.)

Barren sensations come in several varieties. In the interests of brevity, I will focus exclusively on one variety – the images that spontaneously loom up in the visual field when one's eyes are closed (hereafter called *closed-eye sensations*). There are two questions about these sensations that I will address.

First, what about our access to closed-eye sensations? Is it as indirect as our access to belief-generating sensations? It seems to me that the answer is no. We do not apprehend closed-eye sensations by inferring their existence from beliefs that are concerned with other matters. In this respect, our apprehension of them is much more similar to our apprehension of pains and other bodily sensations than to our apprehension of belief-generating sensations.

Second, what is the nature of the relationship between closed-eye sensations and belief-generating sensations? It is clear that they are similar in intrinsic properties. Otherwise we would not be inclined to respond to them in the same way. We would not be inclined to use the same terms in describing closed-eye sensations as we do in describing the visually accessible portion of the extramental world. (For example, we would not be inclined to describe an image as an image of a glowing green rectangle.) But if closed-eye sensations are similar to belief-generating sensations, why are they barren? More concretely, what is it about my image of a green rectangle that prevents me from responding to it in exactly the same way as I respond to belief-generating sensations that are produced by green rectangles that exist out there in the extramental portion of reality? Why doesn't it lead me to believe that there is a glowing green rectangle in front of me? It seems reasonable to explain the fact that images are unable to produce such beliefs by saying that they lack certain of the pictorial qualities that are exemplified by belief-generating sensations. It seems reasonable to suppose that belief-generating sensations have intrinsic qualities that correspond to the properties that confer the appearance of three-dimensionality on two-dimensional paintings. Painters employ a number of well-known techniques to convey the impression that objects are at varying distances from the observer: They convey the sense that lines are receding toward the horizon by making the lines converge; they reduce the size of forms that are intended to be seen as further away from the observer; they invest representations of more remote objects with fewer details; and so on. In a phrase, painters endow their canvases with *pictorial depth cues*. It seems reasonable to suppose that belief-generating sensations have properties that are analogs of pictorial depth cues, and that it is these properties (among others) that endow them with their ability to cause us to form beliefs that are directed on the external world. And it also seems reasonable to suppose that closed-eye sensations fail to generate such beliefs precisely because they lack these analogs of pictorial depth cues.

PART FIVE

Other minds

9

Knowledge of other minds

In this chapter I will be concerned with a group of interrelated epistemological problems.

The first of these problems is the traditional problem of other minds.
Let us say that a qualitative characteristic of sensations is an *immediate
quale* if one or more human beings have direct access to it. Now
common sense encourages one to hold that other human beings have
sensations that are more or less similar to one's own, in the sense of
exemplifying immediate qualia that are more or less like the immediate
qualia one's own sensations exemplify. Common sense also encourages
one to hold that the same is true, though to a lesser degree, of the
members of certain biological species that are not too distant from
homo sapiens. Can these beliefs be justified? If so, how? These two
questions constitute the traditional problem of other minds.

Assuming that this first problem admits of a positive solution, in the
sense that it is possible to show that our intuitions about other human
beings and members of neighboring biological species are justified, the
question arises whether it is possible to justify ascriptions of sensations
with immediate qualia (hereafter called *immediate sensations*) to beings
who stand at some remove from ourselves. Is it possible to justify
ascriptions of immediate sensations to members of remote biological
species? Is it possible to justify ascriptions of such sensations to nonbiological androids? Where are the *bounds of sense* – that is, the lines of
demarcation that separate those beings who may justifiably be said to
have immediate sensations from those beings who may not? These
questions constitute the second problem of other minds.

The third problem concerns the beings who lie beyond the bounds of
sense. By definition, we are not justified in ascribing immediate sensations to these beings, but it remains open whether we would be justified
in denying that they have such sensations. Would we be justified? How?

Most of the material in section I of this chapter is excerpted from "In Defense of Type
Materialism," *Synthese* 59 (1984), 295–320.

To appreciate that there are further problems, recall that we have found it necessary to distinguish between two kinds of qualia. In the first place, there are the qualia that are accessible to direct awareness – the qualia that we have just now agreed to call immediate. This group includes the qualitative characteristics of bodily sensations, gustatory sensations, and olfactory sensations. Second, there are qualia that are not accessible to direct awareness. The members of this group, which include the intrinsic characteristics of visual and auditory sensations, may be called *nonimmediate* qualia. Now, among those authors who maintain a robustly realist attitude toward qualia, and who have succeeded in resisting the temptations of functionalism, there is a tendency to overlook the considerations that suggest that visual and auditory qualia are nonimmediate. They tend to write as if all qualia were immediate. This tendency has nowhere been more in evidence than in the literature on other minds. Authors with a realist, nonfunctionalist view of qualia normally write as if all of the questions about other minds are questions about immediate qualia. Because, however, we have found reason to believe that the class of nonimmediate qualia is non-empty, we are obliged to face some additional questions.

What questions? We seem to have intuitions to the effect that the qualitative characteristics of visual and auditory sensations are pretty much the same throughout the class of human beings – or, to be more accurate, we seem to have intuitions to the effect that these characteristics are pretty much the same among those human beings who resemble one another in the relevant physical and behavioral respects, and to the effect that differences in these qualia are proportional to physical and behavioral differences. Moreover, we seem to hold that members of neighboring biological species can have visual and/or auditory sensations, and that the qualitative characteristics of these sensations are similar in some respects to the qualitative characteristics of the visual and auditory sensations of human beings. Can these intuitions be justified? If so, how? These questions constitute the fourth problem of other minds.

This fourth problem is a counterpart of the first. There are in addition two other problems of other minds, problems that are counterparts respectively of the second and third problems. We must ask, "Are we entitled to attribute visual and auditory sensations to any of the beings who differ radically from ourselves?" This is the fifth problem. As for the sixth problem, it concerns beings to whom we are not justified in attributing visual or auditory sensations. We must ask, "Are we entitled to maintain that these beings lack visual and auditory sensations?"

210

These six problems are intrinsically interesting. But also, it is incumbent on us to make some disposition of them in order to complete our assessment of type materialism. According to type materialism, all beings who are similar to oneself in sensory states are also similar to oneself in neural states, and all beings who are similar to oneself in neural states are also similar in sensory states. It follows that we have no epistemic right to embrace type materialism unless it is possible to justify these two claims. But the task of determining whether the claims can be justified coincides with the task of resolving our six problems about other minds.

I

In this section I will respond to the first of our problems by resuscitating the traditional argument from analogy (AA). If I am right, this oft-reviled argument is eminently successful. Once certain basic improvements have been made, it can be seen to be fully capable of doing its job – which, roughly speaking, is to show that one has every right to suppose that other human beings have immediate sensations that are more or less like one's own, and that one has every right to hold a similar view about the members of neighboring biological species.

The locus classicus of AA is the following passage from John Stuart Mill:

> I am conscious in myself of a series of facts connected by a uniform sequence, of which the beginning is modifications of my body, the middle is feelings, the end is outward demeanor. In the case of other human beings I have the evidence of my senses for the first and last links of the series, but not for the intermediate link. . . . I must either believe [other human beings] to be alive, or to be automatons: and by believing them to be alive, that is, by supposing the link to be of the same nature as in the case of which I have experience, and which is in all other respects similar, I bring other human beings, as phenomena, under the same generalizations which I know by experience to be the true theory of my own existence. And in doing so I conform to the legitimate rules of experimental inquiry.[1]

Let us say that this is the traditional version of AA.

Now the traditional version contains many of the necessary ingre-

1 John Stuart Mill, *An Examination of Sir William Hamilton's Philosophy*, 6th edition (London: Longman's, 1889), pp. 243–44.

dients of a successful version, but it will not quite do as it stands. I propose to replace it with the following version:

> When I consider my own conscious experiences, I find that they play essential roles in all of my sensory explorations of the external world, and also that they are causally linked to all or almost all of the patterns of behavior in my behavioral repertoire. Further, I find that many of the sensory explorations and behavioral ventures that depend on my conscious experiences are essential to my physical well-being and survival. And, finally, when I compare my basic sensory and behavioral capacities with those of other people, I find that they are biologically normal, in the sense that they are shared by almost all other members of my species. Hence, probably all other biologically normal members of my species enjoy conscious experiences like my own. Moreover, it is likely that the experiences of such beings are linked to other factors in perceptual processes and to patterns of behavior by laws that are quite similar to the laws I have found to hold in my own case.

The conclusion of this argument refers only to the class of human beings, but it is possible to construct related arguments that lead to analogous conclusions about larger biological categories.

What are the chief differences between the traditional version of AA and this version? One is that this version represents conscious experiences as playing roles in the organism that are biologically essential. In short, it employs the idea of a *biologically essential role*. Second, in stressing the idea of a normal member of a species, it brings to the fore the idea of a *biological kind*. As we will see later on, it is necessary to appeal to both of these features of the new version in defending AA against its critics.

We must now consider some objections.

The first objection begins with the observation that it is impossible to be directly acquainted with the sensations of others. In view of this, we must recognize that it is impossible to check up on the correctness of AA's conclusion by a confirmation procedure that is more direct. But the objection maintains that this feature of AA is a flaw. It maintains that an analogical argument cannot work unless it is logically possible to reach the conclusion of the argument by some other route.

The second objection is clearly and succinctly formulated in the following passage from Jonathan Dancy's *Introduction to Contemporary Epistemology*:

> The argument from analogy supposes that you can construct from your own case a concept of pains which can be felt by others rather than by you. But is it so easy to conceive of a pain which is not hurting you? You have to start from a pain of yours and conceive of there being something like this which hurts but does not hurt you. . . . How can you conceive of something as painful, as hurting, without conceiving of it as hurting you? Surely, in conceiving of something that hurts, you necessarily conceive of it as painful to *you*. Your conception of pains which are not yours is not a conception of something which is like your pain, since it hurts, but which is not one of yours.[2]

According to Dancy, then, it is impossible to derive a concept of pain from experience without representing pains as things that belong to you. Inevitably, your concept of pain will contain the idea of yourself as a constituent. Accordingly, if your concept of pain has been derived from experience, it cannot be used to ascribe sensations to anyone else.

The third objection consists in pointing out that AA is based on a sample with only one member, and in urging that this feature is a fatal flaw. Paul Churchland states this objection forcefully in the following passage:

> [That the] correlations discovered in one's own case also characterize the cases of every other human can therefore be inferred only by way of an inductive leap from the necessarily solitary instance of one's own (possibly atypical) case. The possible justification available for beliefs about the minds of others is therefore at the vanishing point. One is limited to an incorroborable generalization from a single case. In this way do we arrive at scepticism with respect to the content and even the existence of minds other than one's own.[3]

The first objection seems to me to be the weakest and least interesting of the three. This objection charges that AA is shown to be inadequate by the fact that it is impossible to justify its conclusion by giving a second argument of some other type. But this charge is absurd. Why should the strength of a justification of one type depend on the possibility of finding a second justification of a different type? Perhaps the absurdity can best be seen by considering the enterprise of giving deductive justifications. Many important propositions in number the-

---

2 Jonathan Dancy, *Introduction to Contemporary Epistemology* (Oxford: Blackwell, 1985), p. 70.
3 Paul M. Churchland, *Scientific Realism and the Plasticity of Mind* (Cambridge: Cambridge University Press, 1979), p. 90.

ory cannot be proved unless one uses weak mathematical induction or one of its equivalents. Does this show that it is impossible to justify the propositions in question by giving the standard proofs – that is, by proofs involving weak induction and its equivalents?[4]

The main premise of Dancy's argument is the doctrine that it is impossible to derive a concept of pain from experience without representing pains as things that belong to *you*. Although this doctrine evidently has a certain amount of appeal, it appears to have been soundly refuted many years ago by Hume. Hume wrote:

> For my part, when I enter most intimately into what I call *myself*, I always stumble on some particular impression or other, of heat or cold, light or shade, love or hatred, pain or pleasure. I never can catch *myself* at any time without a perception, and never can observe anything but the perception.[5]

According to Hume, then, insofar as a concept of pain is derived from awareness of individual pains, the concept could not possibly refer to the self. We are not aware of the self in being aware of individual pains; we are only aware of the pains. Indeed, there is no such thing as introspective awareness of the self. Unlike our concepts of types of sensations, our concept of the self cannot be obtained by attending to inner phenomena, nor can the concept of any relation, such as the relation *belonging to*, that is capable of linking sensations to the self.

There is an argument that is closely related to Dancy's argument in a widely discussed paper by Norman Malcolm.[6] Like Dancy, Malcolm is concerned to establish the following proposition: If a sensory concept is derived from introspective awareness of one's own sensations, it isn't possible to use that concept to ascribe sensations to others. However, Malcolm's main premise is somewhat different than Dancy's. Instead of asserting that it is necessary to make use of your concept of yourself in forming a concept of pain, Malcolm asserts that the pains that serve as

---

4 In a valuable paper on AA, Alec Hyslop and Frank Jackson distinguish a number of versions of the first objection and give persuasive replies to all of them. (See Hyslop and Jackson, "The Analogical Inference to Other Minds," *American Philosophical Quarterly* 9 (1972), pp. 168–76. Hyslop and Jackson also give a reply to the third objection that overlaps with my reply. However, they seem not to appreciate the relevance of an idea that I believe to be crucial – the notion of a biological kind. (I am indebted to Michael de Armey for this reference.))
5 See David Hume, *A Treatise of Human Nature*, L.A. Selby-Bigge (ed.) (Oxford University Press, 1967), 251–52.
6 See Norman Malcolm, "Wittgenstein's *Philosophical Investigations*," in Malcolm's *Knowledge and Certainty* (Englewood Cliffs, NJ: Prentice Hall, 1963), pp. 96–129.

the basis for your acquisition of a concept of pain have the property of belonging to you among their essential characteristics. He then infers that the concept you acquire will inevitably stand for a restriction of the property *being a pain*. Specifically, he infers that the concept will inevitably stand for the property *being a pain that belongs to you*. It is then an easy matter to obtain the conclusion that he is after.

Malcolm writes:

> If I were to learn what pain is from perceiving my own pains then I should, necessarily, have learned that pain is something that exists only when I feel pain. For the pain that serves as my paradigm of pain (i.e., my own) has the property of existing only when *I* feel it. That property is essential, not accidental; it is nonsense to suppose that the pain I feel could exist when I did not feel it. So if I obtain my *conception* of pain from pain that I experience, then it will be part of my conception of pain that *I* am the only being that can experience it.[7]

Unfortunately, this reasoning is badly flawed. As Kripke has pointed out, it presupposes a principle that is subject to counterexamples.[8] Suppose that you live in North America, and that you have encountered several small lakes in exploring the territory in the immediate vicinity of your home. Suppose you want to define a term that will stand for the lakes you have observed and also for all similar bodies of water – that is, for lakes in North America and also for lakes in all other parts of the universe. Now if it is ever the case that a property is an essential property of a particular, then presumably it is an essential property of the lakes in your sample that they are located in North America. Does this mean that you are incapable of reaching your goal? Does it mean that you are incapable of introducing a term for the property *being a lake*, and can hope only to introduce a term for the property *being a lake in North America*? Obviously not! Despite the fact that all of the lakes in your sample are located in North America, and despite the fact that this property is probably an essential characteristic of the members of your sample, you can still arrange for your term to stand for the property *being a lake*.

After responding to Malcolm's argument, Kripke goes on to attempt to provide new support for Malcolm's conclusion by constructing an argument of his own. This new argument runs as follows:

---

7 Ibid., pp. 105–06.
8 See Saul A. Kripke, *Wittgenstein on Rules and Private Language* (Cambridge, MA: Harvard Press, 1982), p. 116.

Now the basic problem in extending talk of sensations from 'myself' to 'others' ought to be manifest. Supposedly, if I concentrate on a particular toothache or tickle, note its qualitative character, and abstract from particular features of time and place, I can form a concept that will determine when a toothache or tickle comes again. . . . How am I supposed to extend this notion to the sensations of 'others'? What is this supposed to mean? If I see ducks in Central Park, I can imagine things which are 'like these' – here, still *ducks* – except that they are *not* in Central Park. I can similarly 'abstract' even from *essential* properties of these particular ducks to entities like these but lacking the properties in question – ducks of different parentage and biological origin, ducks born in a different century, and so on. . . . But what can be meant by something 'just like this toothache, only it is not I, but someone else, who has it'? In what ways is this supposed to be similar to the paradigmatic toothache on which I concentrate my attention, and in what ways dissimilar? We are supposed to imagine another entity, similar to 'me' – another 'soul,' 'mind' or 'self' – that 'has' a toothache *just like* this toothache, except that it (he? she?) 'has' it, just as 'I have' this one. All this makes little sense, given the Humean critique of the notion of the self that Wittgenstein accepts. I have no idea of a 'self' in my own case, let alone a generic concept of a 'self' that in addition to 'me' includes 'others'. . . . What are we supposed to abstract from this situation to form the concept of an event which is like the given paradigm case of "it toothaches", except that the toothache is not "mine", but "someone else's"? I have no concept of a 'self' . . . to enable me to make the appropriate abstraction from the original paradigm.[9]

Kripke is here imagining a subject who is confronted with a set of pains, where all members of the set have the property *belonging to myself* as an essential characteristic. The subject is faced with the task of forming a concept that will apply to pains that have this characteristic and also to pains that lack it. To reach this goal, the subject must "abstract away" from the property, and to perform this abstraction, he or she must employ a concept of self. However, given Hume's critique of concept of self, it is dubious that the subject has a concept of self that is equal to the task.

There are two problems with this argument, each of which is sufficient by itself to invalidate it. First, like Malcolm, Kripke appears to be presupposing a principle that is subject to counterexamples. The principle in question comes to this: To abstract away from a property ϕ

9 Ibid., pp. 124–25.

that is an essential characteristic of the members of a certain sample, it is necessary to use a concept that stands for ϕ. To see that this principle is false, observe that it is possible to abstract away from the property *being located in North America* without using a concept that stands for this property. The early American Indians were presumably capable of forming the concept of a lake. To do so they had to abstract away from the property *being located in North America*, for all members of any sample available to them had that property as an essential characteristic. But it is most unlikely that the early Indians had a concept that stood for the property. Second, Kripke attributes a force to Hume's critique of the notion of self that it simply does not have. To bear the weight assigned to it by Kripke's argument, Hume's critique would have to establish that there is *no* procedure that would produce a concept of self that could be used in constructing a generic concept of pain. But in fact it establishes only that it is impossible to derive a concept of self from the data that are given in introspection. Hume's reasoning has no tendency to show that we cannot derive a serviceable concept of self in some other way.[10]

According to the third objection, it is wrong to base an analogical argument on a sample with a single member. It is clear that this presupposition contains an element of truth: Much of the time, a sample with a single member is extremely misleading. However, there are situations in which samples with one member are extremely reliable guides to truth. Here are two such situations:

> **1.** Looking at the philosophy shelf while browsing in my local bookstore, I find that there are five adjacent copies of a book entitled *Reference and Essence*. I take one copy from the shelf and discover that there is a picture of a top hat and a rabbit on the front cover. Noticing that the spines of the remaining copies are exactly like the spine of the copy in my hand, I wonder whether I can be sure that the same picture appears on the other covers. I am aware that publishers occasionally arrange for two or more

10 For example, Hume's critique has no tendency to undermine the view that we can form a serviceable concept of self by forming a concept of a system with a certain functional organization. I see no reason to doubt that we could make use of a concept of this sort in performing the abstractions that Kripke believes to be necessary components of the process of forming a concept of pain. (Incidentally, the idea that our concept of self may represent the self as a certain kind of functional system suggests that Malcolm and Kripke may be wrong in thinking that it is an essential property of your pains that they belong to you. According to a functionalist theory of the self, what makes something your pain is just that it is a substate of the total state of a system with a certain organization. This is presumably a contingent property of the pain.)

different pictures to appear on the covers of different copies of the same book, that cover pictures are sometimes blurred beyond recognition by printing miscues, and that such pictures are sometimes ruined in the course of packing and shipping. But I also know that occurrences of these three types are extremely rare, and that if an occurrence of the second or third type had taken place in this case, the books would probably (though not necessarily) have been returned to the publisher. So I infer that very likely the remaining four covers have the same puzzling picture as the one in my hand.

2. A new species of aquatic mammals is discovered. Scientists observe a number of these mammals, and reach the conclusion that a certain member of the species, named Max, is normal both with respect to behavior and to all external physical characteristics. When Max's body is dissected after his death, they find that it contains two lungs that are roughly equal in size. They calculate that Max's lung capacity was perfectly suited to his patterns of behavior – that is to say, they calculate that if Max had had a larger or smaller capacity, his behavior would have been quite different. They conclude that all normal members of Max's species have two lungs of roughly the same size.

The strength of these arguments is due in part to the nature of the types of resemblance that are seen to link the samples to the larger populations to which the conclusions refer, and it is due in part also to the relationship between these types of resemblance and the properties that are projected over the populations by the conclusions. Thus, in each case, the type of resemblance involved is known to be an extremely reliable sign that objects share all of the properties that belong to a given category, and the property projected by the conclusion is known to belong to the category in question. In short, both arguments satisfy the *reliability condition*. When this condition is not satisfied, larger samples are needed. But when it is satisfied, small samples are entirely legitimate.

Although it seems that this point about sample size is not widely appreciated among philosophers of mind, there are occasional references to it in works by logicians. It is pretty clear, for example, that Frege had something like it in mind while writing the following passage:

> The procedure of the sciences, with its objective standards, will at times find a high probability established by a single confirmatory instance, while at others it will dismiss a thousand as almost worthless. . . .[11]

11 Gottlob Frege, *The Foundations of Arithmetic* (New York: Harper Torchbooks, 1960), p. 16.

We find another version of the point in Copi's elementary logic text:

> An argument based on a single relevant analogy connected with a single instance will be more cogent than one which points out a dozen *irrelevant* points of resemblance between its conclusion's instance and over a score of instances enumerated in its premises.[12,13]

It is clear, I think, that the reliability condition is satisfied by the foregoing version of AA. The population mentioned in the conclusion is known to resemble the sample in that all the elements of both sets are known to be normal members of a single natural kind. Moreover, the following is known to hold: The relation *being normal members of the same natural kind* is a reliable sign that similar overt characteristics are due to similar underlying mechanisms, provided that the characteristics are shared by most of the other members of the kind in question. The situation is somewhat more complex in the case of biological kinds, for there tends to be considerable intraspecific variation even with respect to properties of basic mechanisms. However, although mechanisms of the same type may differ considerably from one another, it is nonetheless true (and known to be true) that different individuals tend to have mechanisms of the same type. Moreover, this is especially true in the case of mechanisms that underlie capacities and behavioral patterns that are essential to physical well-being and survival. Because the contribution of consciousness to physical well-being and survival is on a par with the contributions of breathing, digestion, and circulation of the blood, it is fair to say that projection of qualia is authorized by the reliability condition.[14]

12 Irving M. Copi, *Introduction to Logic*, 5th edition (New York: Macmillan, 1978), p. 338.

13 There is a helpful discussion of the importance of sample size in P. Thagaard and R.E. Nisbett, "Variability and Confirmation," *Philosophical Studies* 42 (1982), pp. 379–94. The arguments in this paper support the position taken here.

14 My argument that the reliability condition is satisfied turns on the claim that the following proposition is known to be true: Essential internal states and mechanisms of beings that belong to the same species tend to be similar in type. This may seem to imply that the foregoing version of AA can only be used by those who have mastered a certain amount of modern biology, but in fact my claim implies nothing of the sort. Notice, for example, that the proposition is strongly supported by the fact that the process that brings any one member of a species into existence is virtually the same as the process by which all of the other members come into existence. One can be fully and vividly aware of this fact without knowing any of the laws that belong to biological theory.

It appears, then, that we are justified in ascribing sensations with immediate qualia to our fellow human beings and to members of neighboring species. But are we justified in ascribing them to beings who lie outside this sphere? I will argue that the answer to this question should be negative.

I will begin by making several observations about our intuitions concerning justification.

First, it seems that most of us feel that we are not entitled to ascribe immediate sensations to members of remote species. Thus, for example, most of us feel fairly confident that we are not entitled to ascribe such sensations to slugs.

Second, as far as I know, almost everyone who has considered the question has fairly deep reservations about attributing immediate sensations to Blockean homunculi-headed robots. Most of us feel that an attribution of this sort would be entirely lacking in justification. Moreover, although there are a few diehard analytic functionalists who claim that we have an epistemic right to make such attributions, it is my impression that these individuals show little enthusiasm for this claim. When they make the claim, they do so with an air of resignation, as if they were discharging a painful duty.

Third, as I maintained in Chapter 3, it is pretty clear that if it had turned out that the brains of human beings were composed of homunculi, our intuitions about Blockean robots would have been quite different. Instead of being reluctant to ascribe immediate sensations to them, we would have insisted on the appropriateness of making such ascriptions.

In combination, these observations make a case for a conclusion that can be expressed as follows: We do not feel justified in ascribing immediate sensations to other beings unless we have reason to believe that the beings in question are biologically similar to ourselves. If the beings are similar to us in structure and composition, we feel justified in ascribing immediate sensations to them. Otherwise we do not.

Before we can commit ourselves to this conclusion fully, however, we must take note of a consideration that seems prima facie to count against it. Although many of us feel that we are not justified in ascribing immediate sensations to silicon-based androids, there is a rather large contingent of professional and lay philosophers who profess to have the opposite intuition. Moreover, when these individuals state their position, they do not do so with an air of embarrassment or resignation. Instead of giving the impression that they feel they are discharging a painful duty, they seem to feel confident that they are entirely right.

No doubt there really are two groups of conflicting intuitions about silicon-based androids, and it may be that there is no way of effecting a reconciliation of the owners of these intuitions – say, by explaining the members of one of the groups away. If so, the philosophy of mind will see a permanent schism. The members of each camp will have a job to do – namely, the job of articulating their own epistemic intuitions, the point being to reach an account of justification that is at least acceptable to themselves. (Those who are not convinced by the line of thought in the next three paragraphs should view this section and the next section as an effort of this sort.) But no one will be qualified to speak for everyone, and there will be no such thing as the correct account of justification.

As I urged at some length in Chapter 3, however, it seems that it is possible to effect a reconciliation here, for it seems that it is possible to explain away the perception that we are justified in attributing immediate sensations to silicon-based androids. This explanation runs as follows: When we reflect on such androids, as we are invited to do every day by novelists, film makers, and prophets, we find that we are inevitably drawn into using the vocabulary of folk psychology in explaining their (imaginary!) behavior. This naturally leads us to think that we are fully justified in applying our sensory terms – in their normal senses – to the internal states of such androids. However, as can be seen by reflecting on Blockean homunculi-heads, this by no means follows. It is no less inevitable that we use sensory terms in explaining the behavior of Blockean homunculi-heads than that we use them in explaining the behavior of silicon-chip-heads. However, it is pretty clear – to most of us, anyway – that it is necessary either to take an instrumentalist attitude in evaluating the former explanations, or to view them as involving an extended, metaphorical use of our sensory terms. No ascription of an immediate sensation to a Blockean homunculi-head is literally correct.

According to the explanation, then, the intuition that we are justified in ascribing sensations to chip-heads rests on a confusion. The intuition is due to the fact that we frequently encounter chip-heads (or similar figures) in imagination, and to the fact that we inevitably respond to them by giving explanations of their behavior that involve

the sensory vocabulary of folk psychology. The intuition arises because
it is easy to confuse the idea that it is necessary to use sensory terms in
explaining the behavior of chip-heads with the idea that we are justified in using sensory terms – in their normal senses – in giving such
explanations. It is easy to see how one could overlook the differences
between these ideas. However, at a deeper level, the differences are
substantial, and there can be no doubt that it would be a mistake to
suppose that the former idea gives us a good reason to think that the
latter idea is correct.

So, it seems, it is possible to explain the intuition away. Ought we to
explain it away? Yes. As we noticed earlier, it seems that we would
have been willing to ascribe sensations to homunculi-heads if our own
brains had turned out to consist of homunculi. We want to embrace the
best explanation of this fact, and it is pretty clear that the best
explanation is the hypothesis that our intuitions about immediate sensations are largely anthropocentric (in the sense that we are guided by
perceived degrees of similarity to ourselves in deciding whether to
ascribe immediate sensations to other beings). However, we cannot
accept this hypothesis if we take the intuition about chip-heads at face
value, for chip-heads are as different from us as homunculi-heads.
Accordingly, the best explanation principle gives us a reason for not
taking the intuition about chip-heads at face value – that is, a reason for
explaining the intuition away.

In view of these considerations, I am inclined to think that our
original picture of our epistemic intuitions was essentially correct.
That is, I am inclined to think that insofar as our epistemic intuitions
are free from distortion and confusion, it is true that we do not feel
justified in ascribing immediate sensations to other beings unless we
have reason to believe that the beings are similar to ourselves in
structure and material composition.

We have now reached a tentative conclusion concerning our intuitions about justification. However, our original goal was not to determine whether we feel that we are justified in ascribing immediate
sensations to beings who are quite different from ourselves, but to
determine whether we really are justified in making such ascriptions.
We originally set out to answer a question about objective justification.
Is there any connection between the conclusion we have reached and
our original goal? Have we made any progress at all?

We have. Consider the following hypothesis about objective justification: AA and its equivalents provide our only real justification for

ascribing immediate sensations to other beings. According to this hypothesis, if an ascription is warranted by AA or an equivalent argument, one is objectively justified in making it. And if an ascription isn't warranted by AA or an equivalent argument, one isn't objectively justified in making it. We are now in a position to see that this hypothesis is compatible with all of our intuitions about justification. (To be more accurate, it is compatible with all of our intuitions about justification that are free from distortion and confusion. I will omit this qualification in the sequel.) Thus, it is compatible with those of our intuitions that refer to other human beings and to members of neighboring species. For each of us has compelling intuitions to the effect that such beings have immediate sensations that are more or less similar to one's own; and, as we saw in the previous section, these intuitions are sustained by AA. It is also compatible with those of our intuitions that refer to beings who are different from us in structure and/or composition. Thus, as we have just seen, these intuitions are negative: We feel that we are not justified in ascribing sensations to beings of the sort in question. And the hypothesis agrees with these feelings. Because it implies that AA is our only justification for ascribing immediate sensations, it implies that we are only justified in ascribing them to beings who are similar to ourselves in respects that can be seen to be highly relevant to the occurrence of our own sensations.

Should we accept this hypothesis? Our intuitions about justification are *our* intuitions, and we are therefore compelled to take them seriously in attempting to answer questions about objective justification. (Our goal in attempting to answer such questions is to find answers which, at the deepest level, make sense to us. It is evident that we must look to our intuitions for guidance if we are to have any hope of success in this enterprise.) This is not to say that we should allow our conclusions about objective justification to be dictated by intuitions. Our intuitions may be confused at certain points (as we have seen), or it may happen that some of them are in conflict with others (which is, in effect, what the skeptic alleges), or there may be some other reason for distrusting them. Rather, the point is that there is always a prima facie case for supposing that an intuition is correct, or, in other words, that we should take an intuition to be correct unless there is some special reason for not doing so.

It seems, then, that we should conclude, albeit tentatively, that the hypothesis is correct. But this conclusion gives us an answer to our original question. It implies that we are not justified in ascribing immediate sensations to members of remote species or to androids. More generally, it implies that we are not justified in ascribing immediate sensations to a being unless the being is similar to ourselves in structure and composition.

Because the notions of structural and compositional similarity are extremely vague, these results tell us very little about the exact location of the line that separates the beings who may justifiably be said to have immediate sensations from the beings who may not. It seems unlikely, however, that it is possible to improve on the results by a philosophical argument. To locate the line of demarcation, we would have to make use of fairly definite information concerning the structure and composition of those components of human beings that are most relevant to the occurrence of immediate sensations. And, of course, philosophy has no special access to such information. Thus, after it has provided the foregoing result, philosophy has no real contribution to make to the task of drawing a line of demarcation. The remaining portions of the task must be turned over to psychophysics and zoology.

III

This brings us to the problem of whether we have an epistemic right to *deny* that beings who are radically different from ourselves are capable of having immediate sensations. In my judgment, we are not in a position today to answer this with a categorical "yes" or a categorical "no." However, as I will now show, we are in a position to endorse the following hypothetical claim: If it is true that there is a correlation between immediate qualia and neural state-types in the case of human beings, then, at such time as the existence of this correlation becomes apparent to us, we will be entitled to answer the problem with a categorical "yes."

Suppose it is true that we will eventually find grounds for believing that there is a correlation between immediate qualia and neural state-types in the case of human beings. Now, assuming that the line of thought of the previous section is correct, we are only justified in ascribing immediate sensations to other beings insofar as there is reason to believe that they are similar to us in the structural and compositional characteristics that are relevant to the occurrence of immediate sensations in us. Hence, on the assumption that we will eventually find grounds for believing that there is a correlation between immediate qualia and other state-types in the case of human beings, we will not be justified in ascribing immediate sensations to beings other than humans unless there is reason to believe that the beings have brain processes that exemplify some of the neural state-types that are exemplified by human brain processes. That is to say, we will never have strong grounds for supposing that the beings in a certain group have sensations that exemplify the immediate quale ϕ unless we also have strong grounds for supposing that the beings have brain processes that exemplify ψ, where ψ is the neural state-type that is correlated with ϕ in the human case.[15]

Thus, if we find that there is a correlation between immediate qualia and neural state-types in the human case, it will inevitably be true that all of our evidence is compatible with the hypothesis that the correlation is universal. By the same token, it will also be true that all of our evidence is compatible with the hypothesis that immediate qualia are identical with neural state-types. But then, it seems, we will have a right to embrace the latter hypothesis if it is the best explanation of the available data. Further, assuming that the line of thought in section II of Chapter 2 is sound, this hypothesis will be the best explanation of the data. So we will have a right to embrace it.

In sum, if it turns out that there is a correlation between immediate qualia and neural state-types in the case of human beings, we will be entitled to accept the thesis that immediate qualia are identical with neural state-types. Now of course, this thesis implies that a being must be similar to us in order to have immediate sensations. So we have the promised result: If it turns out that there is a correlation between immediate qualia and neural state-types in the case of human beings, then, at such time as this correlation becomes apparent to us, we will be entitled to deny that beings who are radically different from ourselves are capable of having immediate sensations.

IV

We must now turn to consider our three problems about nonimmediate qualia and the sensations that exemplify them. These are: first, the problem of whether we are justified in making more or less uniform

15 This claim does not imply that we will never have strong grounds for attributing immediate sensations to members of other biological species. This is because, as we observed earlier, certain of the principles of individuation that are used in neuroscience determine state-types that are highly inclusive.

ascriptions of nonimmediate sensations to human beings and to members of neighboring species; second, the problem of whether we have a right to ascribe nonimmediate sensations to beings who are different from ourselves; and third, the problem of whether we have a right to deny that the latter beings are capable of having nonimmediate sensations.

Because our concepts of nonimmediate qualia owe their existence to the laws of folk psychology, the task of determining which uses of the concepts are justified requires us to consider the content and epistemic status of these laws. Now the laws imply that human beings who are similar in the relevant physical respects are also similar in nonimmediate sensations, and that differences in nonimmediate sensations are proportional to physical differences. Hence, if we are justified in accepting the laws of folk psychology, we are also justified in holding that human beings tend to be similar in nonimmediate sensations in proportion to their relevant physical similarities. And it would seem that we are justified in accepting the laws of folk psychology. For folk psychology enjoys a great deal of predictive and explanatory success, and this success argues forcefully for the proposition that its picture of the workings of the human mind is more or less correct.[16]

What about members of neighboring species? Are we justified in holding that they have nonimmediate sensations that are proportionally similar to the nonimmediate sensations of human beings? And what about beings who are quite different from ourselves? Are we justified in ascribing nonimmediate sensations to them?

To answer these questions, we must return to the conclusions we reached in Chapters 7 and 8. We observed that our concepts of nonimmediate qualia are both complex and variegated, but that they all have constituents (for example, the concept of a sensation) whose referents are fixed by folk psychological descriptions. These descriptions constrain their respective concepts to refer to the state-types that play certain functional roles in human beings. It follows that we are justified in using our concepts of nonimmediate qualia in connection with other beings only insofar as we have independent reason to believe that the other beings are capable of being in states that exemplify these state-types. It follows from this in turn that we are entitled to ascribe nonimmediate sensations to beings who are relevantly similar to our-

16 This little argument is intended as an abbreviated version of the line of thought in Chapter 1 of Jerry Fodor's *Psychosemantics* (Cambridge, MA: M.I.T. Press, 1987).

selves, and that we are not entitled to ascribe them to beings who are not relevantly similar to ourselves.

Is it appropriate to deny that beings who are quite different from ourselves are capable of having nonimmediate sensations? Once again we are only in a position to give a hypothetical answer. If it should turn out that there are neural state-types that play the functional roles in human beings that are assigned to nonimmediate qualia by folk psychology, we will have a fact that is badly in need of explanation (namely, the fact that certain neural state-types and certain qualia occupy the same functional roles in human beings), and, by the same token, we will have a best explanation argument for the claim that nonimmediate qualia are identical with neural state-types. Because this claim implies the proposition that nonimmediate qualia do not have instances in beings who are quite different than ourselves, our best explanation argument for the claim will give us a right to accept this proposition.

10

Unity of consciousness, other minds, and phenomenal space

In this chapter I will present and defend a theory of unity of consciousness. The theory that I will recommend has two features that set it apart from other theories about the same topic. First, it asserts that it is a mistake to think of unity of consciousness as having just one source. There are a number of different relations (hereafter called *unity relations*) that count as sources or forms of unity of consciousness. Second, my theory denies that all of the sources or forms of unity are *compositional*. Let us say that a relation R is compositional if it meets two conditions: First, the relata of R are sensations; second, there exists some other relation R' such that if x and y stand in the relation R to one another, they do so because x and y both bear R' to some other thing that is not itself a sensation. For example, *having the same owner as* is compositional: When two sensations bear this relation to one another, they do so because each of them stands in the relation *being owned by* to the same subject of experience. A relation is *purely sensory* if its relata are sensations and it is not compositional. I will defend the view that some unity relations are purely sensory. In presenting my theory of unity, it will prove convenient to have a term for the binary relation R such that two sensations bear R to each other if and only if they are members of an array of sensations that exhibits some form or other of unity of consciousness. *Co-consciousness* is the term that I will use. (In effect, then, "co-consciousness" will be a term for the disjunctive relation consisting of all members of the class of binary unity relations.)

Questions about the unity of consciousness are intrinsically interesting, but this is not my only reason for pursuing them here. It is necessary to identify the factors that make for unity of consciousness in

Although my views about unity of consciousness diverge sharply from his views, I have benefited deeply from conversations with Ivan Fox. I have also been helped considerably by advice from Louise Antony, Joseph Levine, and David Westendorf.

order to understand fully a distinction that is presupposed in the previous chapter – the distinction between your mind and mine. The unity of my consciousness is a condition of the possibility of our being able to draw this distinction in a meaningful way.

I

It is initially tempting to think that unity of consciousness should be analyzed exclusively in terms of ownership – that being co-conscious should be identified with the relation *being owned by the same subject of experience as*. But this view quickly loses much of its initial appeal. Although it is arguably the case that *being owned by the same subject of experience as* is one of the main sources or forms of unity of consciousness, it is certainly not the only one.

To see this, consider the relation *being next to*. It is clear that it is a unity relation: If two sensations are next to each other in the sensory field (in the way in which, say, a sensation of pressure in my thumb can be next to another sensation of pressure in my thumb), they fulfill the requirements of our intuitive notion of co-consciousness. It is also clear that *being next to* is not the same relation as *being owned by the same subject of experience as*. Thus, although sensations bear the former relation to one another by virtue of their positions in the sensory field, they bear the latter relation to one another by virtue of standing in the relation *belonging to* to some third entity. The relations have different properties.

In claiming that *being next to* and *being owned by the same subject as* are both unity relations, I mean to claim that they are independent sources of unity. Against this view, it might be said that *being next to* implies *being owned by the same subject as*, and that the former somehow derives its power to unify sensations from this fact. However, this objection is both unfair and misguided. The objection is unfair because it is not at all clear that *being next to* implies *being owned by the same subject as*. Thus, it seems to be conceptually possible for there to be a pair of sensations that are not owned by anyone, but that are nevertheless linked by the relation *being next to*. And if it is conceptually possible for there to be a pair of sensations of this sort, perhaps it is logically possible as well. The objection is misguided because, even if *being next to* implies *being owned by the same subject as*, it is still not true that the former owes its power to unify sensations to the latter. *Caeteris paribus*, sensations that are owned by the same subject and that are next to each other in phenomenal space are unified in a different way, and also count intui-

229

tively as being more unified, than sensations that are owned by the same subject but that are spatially discrete.

The ownership theory errs in claiming that *being owned by the same subject as* is the only form of unity of consciousness. But would it be correct to say that this relation is *one* of the forms of unity? It seems fair to say that we have intuitions that favor a positive answer. However, before accepting this answer, we must examine an objection.

Parfit tries to justify a negative answer by appealing to a case of brain bisection.[1] In the example he describes, all of a certain man's memories, psychological capacities, and personality traits are stored in each of his two hemispheres. (It is of course dubious that Mother Nature would ever arrange for such a duplication, but Parfit is concerned only to describe a case that is logically possible.) The man is equipped with a device that can block communication between hemispheres, and this device is within his control. So as to be able to try out two ways of approaching a physics problem simultaneously, he activates the device for a period of ten minutes. Each of the hemispheres is able to remember all that has previously happened to him; and when communication is restored at the end of ten minutes, he can remember all of the psychological states that have been associated with each of the hemispheres during the interval. However, while they are disconnected, neither of the hemispheres has direct access to the psychological states of the other. Each of them stands in much the same epistemic relation to the psychological states of the other as normal persons do to the psychological states of other normal persons.

Parfit seems to recognize that we have some temptation to describe this case as one in which one man is temporarily replaced by two men, but he urges that it is best seen as a case in which one man has two streams of consciousness. He writes: "Given the brief and modest nature of this disunity, it is not plausible to claim that this case involves more than a single person."[2] Because he interprets the case in this way, he is able to view it as a counterexample to the claim that ownership by the same man is a sufficient condition of co-consciousness.

Parfit's line of thought is not convincing. He thinks that the brevity of the interval during which the hemispheres are disconnected is a reason for maintaining that the original man remains in existence

---

1 See Derek Parfit, *Reasons and Persons* (Oxford: Oxford University Press, 1984), pp. 246–48.
2 Ibid., p. 248.

during the interval (and that no other man exists during the interval). But this is wrong. What makes something a man is not his life expectancy but rather the fact that he is sentient and has a certain functional organization. Moreover, it is simply false to say that the disunity is modest: There are two distinct streams of consciousness, two distinct cognitive systems, two distinct sets of motives and goals, and so on. The subjects housed in the different hemispheres are of course similar, but similarity between two subjects is hardly a good reason for asserting that they constitute a single subject.

II

Another standard view about unity of consciousness is summarized clearly in the following passage from Parfit's *Reasons and Persons*:

> The unity of consciousness does not need a deep explanation. It is simply a fact that several experiences can be *co-conscious*, or be the objects of a single state of awareness. It may help to compare this fact with the fact that there is short-term memory of what is called 'the specious present'. Just as there can be a single memory of just having had several experiences, such as hearing a bell strike three times, there can be a single state of awareness both of hearing the fourth striking of this bell, and of seeing raven fly past the bell-tower. Reductionists claim that nothing more is involved in the unity of consciousness at a single time. Since there can be one state of awareness of several experiences, we need not explain this unity by ascribing these experiences to the same person, or subject of experiences.[3]

According to this second account, then, two sensations are constituents of the same state of consciousness if they are the objects of a single state of introspective awareness. But this proposition is only the core idea. In order to do justice to the facts, it is necessary to add a couple of embellishments. One relevant fact is that sensations can be co conscious even when they are not objects of actual states of awareness. Consider the last time you were aware of a pain. Probably you also had a number of visual sensations at the time – let us suppose that one was a case of phenomenal blue. You may well have been aware of the external patch of blue that was represented by your visual sensation; but if the case was typical, you probably were not aware of the sensation itself. (You did not explicitly believe that you were then having a sensation that exemplified phenomenal blue.) In order to accommodate cases of

---

3 Ibid., pp. 250–51.

231

this sort, the theory must analyze co-consciousness in terms of potential states of awareness. There are not enough actual states of awareness to meet the theory's requirements. Second, it is evident that myriads of sensations can be co-conscious at a single moment. This suggests that it is possible – even likely – that the number of co-conscious sensations can exceed the number of sensations that can be objects of a single state of awareness. Accordingly, it would probably be a mistake to claim that a set of sensations is co-conscious just in case all of the members of the set can be the objects of a single state of awareness. Instead, the theory should claim that the members of the set are co-conscious just in case they can be brought together pairwise by states of awareness.

When the relevant facts have been taken into account and the appropriate embellishments have been made, we wind up with a version of the awareness theory that looks like this: Where S is a set of simultaneously occurring sensations, it is necessarily the case that the members of S are constituents of the same state of consciousness if and only if, for every pair of members x and y of S, x and y can be objects of a single state of introspective awareness.

Like the ownership theory, the awareness theory contains an element of truth. For surely it is correct to say that sensations show a certain unity or togetherness if they are, or can be, objects of the same state of introspective awareness. However, although it is true that the awareness theory correctly identifies one of the sources or forms of unity, it is also true that the theory errs in claiming that it is the only source.

To see this, notice first that there are lower animals who appear to have unified sensory fields but who do not display the sort of conceptual sophistication that a being must have in order to be capable of having introspective beliefs. Consider raccoons. It is plausible to say that raccoons have visual sensations, and it is also plausible to say that they have beliefs. But can raccoons have beliefs about visual sensations? Can they form concepts that stand for various phenomenal shapes and phenomenal colors? We have no reason to think that the answer is positive, and considerations of simplicity favor a negative answer.

Further, the awareness theory implies that when one is aware of one's sensory field as unified, one is either aware that one's sensations are actually the objects of a single state of awareness, or aware that they are capable of becoming such objects. It implies, in other words, that awareness of unity of consciousness is a form of second-order awareness. This may well be correct in some cases, but there are plenty of cases in which it fails to hold. When I am aware of my sensory field as unified, it seems to me that I am aware of the existence of a number of individual sensations, and it also seems that I am aware that these sensations are intimately related to one another. But it does not always seem that I am aware of a state of awareness, and still less does it always seem that I am aware of a relational fact involving a state of awareness and my individual sensations. In short, the awareness theory is at variance with the phenomenology of awareness of unity.

Finally, it is possible to argue constructively against the awareness theory by adverting to *being owned by the same subject of experience as* and *being next to*. As we noticed earlier, these two relations are unity relations. Because they are clearly different relations than *being an object of the same state of awareness as*, it must be wrong to identify co-consciousness with the latter relation.

III

A third account of unity of consciousness is suggested by the following passage from a recent monograph by Sydney Shoemaker.

> [The] functionalist account of mind has implications concerning the synchronic unity of minds. It is only when the belief that it is raining and the desire to keep dry are copersonal that they tend (in conjunction with other mental states) to lead to such effects as the taking of an umbrella; if the belief is mine and the desire is yours, they will not directly produce any joint effects. And it seems that if a belief and desire do produce (in conjunction with other mental states) just those effects which the functional characterizations of them say they ought to produce if copersonal, then in virtue of this they are copersonal. We can make sense of the idea that a single body might be simultaneously 'animated' by two different minds or consciousnesses; the phenomena that would make it reasonable to believe that this had happened would be similar to, but more extreme than, the phenomena observed in 'split-brain' patients that have led some investigators to think that splitting the brain results in splitting the mind. Whether different mental states that are realized in such a body should count as belonging to the same person, or mind, would seem to turn precisely on whether they are so related that they will jointly have the functionally appropriate sorts of effects.[4]

Shoemaker is here concerned with a grander topic than the one we are presently considering. His topic is the synchronic unity of a person, and

---

4 See Sydney Shoemaker and Richard Swinburne, *Personal Identity* (Oxford: Blackwell, 1984), p. 94.

ours is the unity of a state of consciousness. But his remarks suggest an interesting account of the latter. This account may be expressed by saying that the relation *being co-conscious* should be identified with the relation *jointly having the functionally appropriate sort of effects*. That is to say, according to this account, it is necessary that two sensations are co-conscious if and only if together they have causal and counterfactual properties that neither has alone, and by virtue of these properties they can be said to have produced or to be capable of producing a number of "appropriate" psychological and behavioral effects. (Co-conscious sensations often stand in causal and counterfactual relations to each other in addition to standing in such relations to other things. Thus, it is generally true of each member of a pair of itches that if it were to gain considerably in point of intensity, the intensity of the other would decrease. Facts of this sort would have to be included in any list of appropriate psychological and behavioral effects.)

Like its predecessors, the functionalist theory calls attention to an important member of the family of unity relations. It is natural to think of sensations as being parts of a unified system if they are capable of joining together to carry forward the essential business of the system. However, again like its predecessors, the functionalist theory makes the mistake of claiming that there is only one unity relation.

We can argue constructively against the functionalist theory by appealing to *being owned by the same subject of experience as, being next to*, and *being an object of the same state of awareness as*. As we have seen, all three of these relations are forms of unity of consciousness. Moreover, because they are all distinct from one another, it cannot be true that the relation *jointly having the functionally appropriate sort of effects* is identical with all of them. So there are at least two forms of unity of consciousness that the functionalist theory fails to capture.

Perhaps a functionalist will reply as follows: "There are a number of different functional relations that count as forms of unity of consciousness, and it is therefore a mistake to think of the expression 'jointly having the functionally appropriate sort of effects' as standing for a single relation. Actually it stands ambiguously for the members of a family of functional relations, where each member of the family corresponds to a way of replacing 'functionally appropriate sort of effects' with a list of specific types of effect. One member of the family can be identified with *being owned by the same subject as*, a second with *being next to*, and a third with *being an object of the same state of awareness as*."

The main idea here – the idea that there is a whole family of functionally definable unity relations – is a plausible one. However, this reply concedes one of the main points at issue – that there is a plurality of unity relations. Moreover, although I am prepared to acknowledge that *being owned by the same subject as* and *being an object of the same state of awareness as* are functional relations, I think that this is clearly false of *being next to*. *Being next to* is a counterpart of such qualitative monadic properties as *being a pain* and *being an itch*. This can be seen by observing that it is possible to construct arguments concerning *being next to* that are like the ones that were used in Chapter 3 to discredit the functionalist accounts of *being a pain* and its fellows. Here, for example, is a short argument concerning *being next to* that is inspired by the first heterogeneity argument: Just as it appears to be nomologically possible for a being with few, if any, cognitive abilities and no behavioral capacities to have a pain (consider the brain of a young baby kept alive in a vat), so also it appears to be nomologically possible for a being with few, if any, cognitive abilities and no behavioral capacities to have two pains that stand in the relation *being next to*; hence, just as the capacity to have pains seems not to depend on the functional states by which it is accompanied in adult humans, so also the capacity to have phenomenally adjacent pains seems not to depend on such states. (In adapting the foregoing antifunctionalist arguments to *being next to* it is necessary to make some changes. This is because *being next to* is a relation rather than a monadic property. However, what is at issue in the foregoing arguments is the question of whether a psychological property is definable in terms of relations of two kinds – causal relations and probabilistic relations. The question of whether a psychological relation is definable in terms of relations of these two kinds is similar to this question, and it should therefore not be surprising that it can be answered by similar arguments.)

IV

There are at least two quite different part-whole relations that have sensations as their relata. As we will soon see, "part" can be used as a term for a relation between sensations that is quite similar to a spatial part-whole relation – that is, to a part-whole relation that takes objects in physical space as its relata. But it is also possible to speak of sensations as parts without making a claim that has any spatial significance. Consider, for example, a sensation that corresponds to a short temporal segment of a performance of a symphony. This sensation may

235

include a sensation corresponding to the note produced by the oboe. If so, the oboe-sensation is a part of the whole-orchestra-sensation. And because auditory sensations are not extended in phenomenal space, the relevant sense of "part" cannot be explained in spatial terms.

Suppose that there is also a sensation corresponding to the note produced by the tuba. This sensation is part of the sensation corresponding to the combined sounds of all the instruments, and this appears to be a sufficient reason for saying that the tuba-sensation is co-conscious with the oboe-sensation. By the same token, it is natural to favor an idea about unity of consciousness that can be expressed as follows: It is necessarily the case that x is co-conscious with y if x and y are parts (in a nonspatial sense of "part") of the same sensation. As is evident from its form, this idea differs from the theories discussed in earlier sections in that it claims only to specify a sufficient condition of unity. There is no point in our continuing to consider theories that claim to identify conditions that are both necessary and sufficient, for we are already in a position to conclude that such theories are false.

This leaves us with the problem of spelling out the content of the present idea by finding an appropriate sense of "part." A natural suggestion is that the appropriate sense can be explained in terms of causation. It seems, for example, that one of the key differences between the tuba-sensation and the whole-orchestra-sensation is that a full causal explanation of the latter is at least implicitly a full causal explanation of the former. Generalizing directly from this example, we can say that it is true, and true as a matter of necessity, that an event x is part of an event y if and only if (1) x occupies the same temporal interval as y, (2) every actual state of affairs that is a causally sufficient condition of y is also a causally sufficient condition of x, and (3) it is not the case that every actual state of affairs that is a causally sufficient conditon of x is a causally sufficient condition of y. A flaw of this explanation is that it prevents us from saying that an event is part of itself. However, we can provide for the desire to say such things by disjoining the conjunction of (1)–(3) with "x is identical with y."

V

Sensations exemplify a number of relations that are analogous to the relations that physical objects exemplify by virtue of their locations in physical space. We have already taken note of a member of this set of p-spatial relations – namely, the relation *being next to*. (Here and else-

236

where, I write "*p*-spatial" as an abbreviation of "phenomenal spatial.") We have observed that *being next to* entails co-consciousness, and we have also observed that this form of co-consciousness is interestingly different from the other forms. We must now take a closer look at the set of *p*-spatial relations.

In addition to *being next to*, the set includes, for example, *being p-spatially near to*, *being a p-spatial part of*, and *being in the same p-spatial place as*. As these examples suggest, the members of the set are all purely phenomenal relations in the sense that it is possible to be introspectively aware of facts in which they are involved. All of them take concrete sensations and *p*-spatial parts of concrete sensations as their relata. And all of them count intuitively as unity relations.[5]

We can use introspection to grasp what it is for one sensation to stand in a *p*-spatial relation to another; and introspection gives us no reason to believe that such facts are in any way more problematic than facts involving phenomenal properties like *being a pain* and *being a bitter gustatory sensation*. Indeed, all things considered, it seems that the former facts are fundamentally similar to the latter. (I should add, in explanation of this point, that the members of the set are all synchronic – they link only sensations and *p*-spatial parts of sensations that occur at the same time.)

Now it can be intuitively correct to say that two sensations are co-spatial even though they do not stand in any of the *p*-spatial relations that we have considered thus far. For example, although a pain in my left hand is co-spatial with an itch in my right hand, the pain cannot be said to be next to the itch, or near the itch, or in the same place as the itch. (To be sure, there is a sense in which it can be said to be near the itch – given that one hand is touching the other. But this sense of "near" is not the one that is relevant here.)

The question therefore arises, "Is there a *p*-spatial relation that connects all of the pairs of sensations and *p*-spatial parts of sensations

---

5 I am strongly inclined to think that expressions like "being *p*-spatially near to" stand ambiguously for two or more relations. Thus, for example, it seems quite unlikely that we are using "near to" in the same sense when we say that a pain is near to an itch as when we say that a sensation in the lower left quadrant of the visual field is near to another sensation in the same quadrant. In general, it seems unlikely that we are using "near to" in the same sense when we are talking about bodily sensations as when we are talking about visual sensations.

It follows that expressions defined in terms of "being *p*-spatially near to," such as "extended synchronic *p*-spatial proximity" (see the antepenultimate section of this paragraph), may well be ambiguous, too.

that fall under our intuitive concept of sensory co-spatiality?" I think that there is in fact a relation that meets this condition. In order to define it we must first introduce the concept of *extended synchronic p-spatial proximity*: Where x and y are two sensations or two p-spatial parts of sensations, x bears *extended synchronic p-spatial proximity* to y if and only if it is possible for there to be a series of sensations such that (1) x and y are the end points of the series, and (2) each member of the series is near to some other point of the series. Once this concept is in hand, sensory co-spatiality can be explained as follows: Where x and y are sensations or p-spatial parts of sensations, x belongs to the same phenomenal space as y if and only if x bears extended synchronic p-spatial proximity to y.

This definition seems to work. Thus, although the pain in my left hand is not connected to the itch in my right hand by a series of actual sensations, it is possible for there to be a series that connects them (that is, it is possible for there to be a series that extends up my left arm, across my chest, and down my right arm). It follows that the pain bears *extended synchronic p-spatial proximity* to the itch. Given our definition, this implies in turn that the pain and the itch are co-spatial. This is exactly the result that our intuitive concept of co-spatiality requires.

I remarked earlier that *being next to, being p-spatially near to, being a p-spatial part of,* and *being in the same p-spatial place as* are all unity relations. What about *extended synchronic p-spatial proximity*? Is it a unity relation? It seems that the answer should be "yes," for it seems that two sensations count intuitively as components of a *system* if they bear this relation to one another. However, it also seems that *extended synchronic p-spatial proximity* makes for a less intimate sort of unity than the other p-spatial relations we have considered. It seems that it confers unity on pairs of sensations, but only unity of a low degree.

VI

We have now considered a number of different relations. They are all relations that meet two conditions: They count as sources or forms of unity of consciousness, and they can be seen to exist from the perspective of psychology. It is tempting to think that they are the *only* relations that meet both of these conditions. But before we can embrace this view we must consider two questions.

First, what about neural relations between sensations? If sensations are identical with brain states, then neuroscience will no doubt be able to call attention to some heretofore unrecognized relations that can be seen to bring sensations into some sort of mutual relevance. Won't these relations belong in the same category as the ones we have already identified? No. Insofar as they are specified in the vocabulary of neuroscience, neural relations cannot be seen to exist from the perspective of psychology. Hence, if a neural relation is not type-identical with a relation that can be seen on independent grounds to be a unity relation, it should not be grouped with the relations that we have already identified.

This is perhaps the place to mention that some of these relations may well turn out to be type-identical with neural relations. To be sure, this is not true of all members of our family of relations: It is clear, for example, that *being capable of becoming an object of the same state of awareness as* is a functional relation. However, it seems that *being next to* and several other members of the same family are qualitative rather than functional in nature. If so, they may well be type-correlated with neural relations. And of course, here as elsewhere, a type-correlation is a good reason for claiming identity.

This brings us to the second question. I have sometimes felt that it is possible to discriminate introspectively a form of co-consciousness that is different from all of the forms that we have considered up to now. Thus, it has sometimes seemed, when I have been focusing on a pair of auditory sensations, or a pair of sensations associated with different sense modalities, that I was directly aware of the sensations as co-conscious even though I was not aware of them as owned by the same subject, nor as objects of a single state of awareness, nor as standing in any causal or counterfactual relations to one another or to something else, nor as parts of some third sensation, nor as linked by some *p*-spatial relation. I have never felt that I was aware of this new form of co-consciousness as having positive differentiae that distinguish it from the other forms. Rather I was aware only that it lacks the positive differentiae that belong respectively to the other forms. Accordingly, it has seemed to me that this form of co-consciousness is pure – that it has no distinguishing characteristics other than its ability to unite sensations.

Although at one point in my reflections on unity of consciousness I was strongly inclined to think that there must be a ghostly form of co-consciousness that answers to this description, I now feel that this view is wrong. It isn't possible to find this ghostly form of co-consciousness within one's experience. Hence, there is no good reason to believe that it exists.

As I now see it, when it seems to me that I am aware of a fact involving two auditory sensations, or two sensations associated with different sense modalities, and a ghostly unity relation, I am only aware of a fact that consists of the simultaneous existence of the two sensations. This is the only fact involving the sensations that is given. If it were otherwise, I would be able to distinguish introspectively between the fact consisting of the simultaneous existence of the two sensations and the fact consisting of the two sensations and the putative ghostly unity relation. There would be a detectable difference between these two facts. However, as can be seen from the very ghostliness of the putative unity relation, there is no such difference. As I now see it, when it seems to me that the co-consciousness of the sensations is an object of awareness, I am making a mistake. I am projecting the unity that is created and sustained by my state of awareness out into the fact of which I am aware. That is to say, I am projecting the Parfitian unity that is brought into existence by my state of awareness out into the fact that serves as the object of my awareness.

VII

Before we bring our reflections on unity of consciousness to a close, we ought to consider the possibility that despite appearances to the contrary, it is a mistake to attempt to view *relations* as the primary source of unity. Consider the difference between a situation that contains two sensations that are united in a single consciousness and a situation that contains two sensations that belong to different consciousnesses. It is extremely tempting to describe this difference by saying that the sensations in the first situation are connected by a relation that is not involved in the second situation. However, there is an alternative account that is suggested by Carnap's *Aufbau* and that has recently been defended by Ivan Fox.[6] According to this other picture, a momentary state of consciousness cannot possibly be said to consist of individual sensations. Indeed, there is no such thing as an individual sensation. Reality can be claimed only for the momentary cross-sections of the stream of experience that count as entire states of consciousness. To borrow a term from Carnap, reality can be claimed only for *elemen-*

---

6 See Rudolf Carnap, *The Logical Structure of the World* (Berkeley and Los Angeles: University of California Press, 1967). Fox's paper, "The Unity of Consciousness and Other Minds," has never been published.

240

tarerlebnesse. When one is in an internal state that seems to involve an individual sensation with a given qualitative character ϕ, one should strictly speaking describe the situation by saying that one's current *elementarerlebnis* has the property *being partly ϕ-ish*, or by saying that it is a member of a certain similarity class of *elementarerlebnesse*. Talk of individual sensations is just a *façon de parler*. Hence, it is wrong to say that the first of our two situations involves three different individuals, a pair of sensations and a state of consciousness of which the two sensations are constituents. Rather it contains just one individual, an *elementarerlebnis*. And by the same token it is wrong to say that the difference between our two situations is the difference between there being two sensations that stand in a certain relation and there being two sensations that do not. Rather it is a special case of the difference between there being a single individual of a given type and there being two individuals of that same type.

This alternate picture of the unity of consciousness suffers from a rather serious flaw. Thus, observe that the alternate account consists of two components: First, there is the proposition that whole states of consciousness are "natural units" or "proper individuals"; second, there is the proposition that sensations are not "proper individuals," and that they can be said to exist only as logical constructions. In order to justify the first component of the alternate picture, one must give reasons for according the status of proper individual to whole states of consciousness. However, there are grounds for thinking that these reasons would also be reasons for according the same status to sensations. Thus, it seems that any defense of the first component would implicitly provide a rationale for rejecting the second component.

When we determine whether it is appropriate to recognize something as a proper individual, we apply a set of general criteria that might be called *principles of entification*. It is possible to get a feeling for the content of the criteria in question by taking note of the common features of the things in the physical world that we regard as proper individuals. Some of these features are captured by the following conditions:

> x has fairly well defined boundaries (in the sense that there are salient and important qualitative differences between x's interior and things that are external to x); (1)

> x is continuous (in the sense that each of x's parts is joined with or contiguous to at least one of its other parts); (2)

241

x's environment can change significantly without depriving x of existence and without changing the qualitative character of x beyond recognition;   (3)

The most proximate causes of x's existence are importantly and saliently different (though not necessarily different in kind) than the most proximate causes of other individuals in x's environment;   (4)

x exhibits a certain amount of qualitative homogeneity;   (5)

x exhibits dynamic cohesiveness (in the sense that its constituents tend to "hang together when subjected to various stresses").[7]   (6)

(1)–(6) are not the only conditions that are normally satisfied by things in the physical world that count as proper individuals. Nor is it the case that every proper individual in the physical world satisfies all of (1)–(6). However, it is reasonable to suppose that (1)–(6) figure importantly in our principles of entification. We are strongly inclined to view something that satisfies all six of the conditions as a proper individual, and we are strongly disinclined to accord that status to something that does not satisfy any of them.

These claims are confirmed by the fact that (1)–(6) tend to be satisfied by sensations as well as by physical objects. To be sure, certain of the key terms (especially "boundary" and "interior") have to be construed somewhat differently in connection with sensations than in connection with physical objects, and in some cases the satisfaction is only vacuous (sensations without parts can be said to satisfy (2) and (6) vacuously). But with these qualifications it seems fair to say that (1)–(6) explain our willingness to count sensations as proper individuals quite well.

(A remark about the relevant senses of "boundary" and "interior": Insofar as one is concerned only to apply these terms to sensations that are extended, they can be said to have senses that are the same, when viewed from a certain level of abstraction, as the senses that they have when they are used to talk about objects that are extended in physical space. But it is necessary to introduce a special convention to cover cases in which they are used in connection with unextended sensations. Here is the obvious candidate: If a sensation is unextended, then

7 The term "dynamic cohesiveness" and my definition of it are borrowed from Eli Hirsch. See Hirsch, *The Concept of Identity* (Oxford: Oxford University Press, 1982), p. 108. My discussion of entification is indebted to Hirsch's discussion at several other points.

"interior" stands for the sensation itself, taken as a whole, and "boundary" has the same reference as "interior.")

Now if an advocate of the alternate picture of the unity of consciousness were to attempt to defend the view that whole states of consciousness are proper individuals, he or she would find it necessary to appeal to our principles of entification. Such an appeal might well be at least partially successful. Thus, for example, although it is not immediately clear what it would mean to speak of the "boundary" or the "environment" of a whole state of consciousness, it seems intuitively appropriate to say that whole states of consciousness can satisfy conditions (1), (3), and (4). However, in appealing to our principles of entification, an advocate of the alternate picture would be implicitly acknowledging their authority to settle disputes about what is to count as a proper individual. And by the same token the advocate would be implicitly granting that it is legitimate to reject the second component of the alternate picture – namely, the claim that sensations are not proper individuals. For as we have just seen, our principles of entification imply that this claim is false.

Index

absent functional role argument (absent role argument), 61–5, 75, 166
absent qualia argument, 57–62, 68, 166; second, 70–3, 77–8
absolute thresholds, 129n10
activation, 118, 121–2, 123, 126
active introspection, 118–22, 123–6
Aeschylus, 147
aesthetic considerations: in justification of type materialism, 40
Albritton, Roger, 128–9
Alzheimer's disease, 62, 74, 150, 151
analytic functionalism, 53–5, 68, 72, 167, 168; ascription of sensations to others, 220; central doctrine of, 55, 165; differences from psychofunctionalism, 55–6; names synonymous with folk-psychological descriptions, 57–67, 70, 75, 165–7, 181
androids, 80, 169; ascription of mental states to, 45; ascription of psychological terms to, 54; ascription of sensations to, 5, 10, 70–3, 77, 167, 181, 209, 220–1; silicon-based, 68, 71–3, 77, 220–1
anthropocentricity, 166, 222
anticipation, 107, 128
anti-realism, 107, 108
Antony, Louise, 228n
appeal to other species, 105–6
appearance/reality distinction, 127, 130
appearances: entertaining, 190–1, 192, 193, 200, 201, 203n10; language of, 198–9, 202; and visual sensations, 203
argument from analogy, 15, 211–19, 222–3
Armey, Michael de, 214n4

Armstrong, David M., 95–6, 96n11, 98n12, 119n2, 127, 127n9, 164n1
ascription of mental states, 45
attention, 119, 120, 123, 124–6
attribute-identity bridge laws, 24n5
auditory perception, 189
auditory sensations, 138, 239–40; in phenomenal space, 236; qualitative characteristics of, 210
aversion to pain, 74–5, 77, 78, 79
awareness: of belief-generating sensations, 187–206; of mental states, 95–7; of sensations, 12; of visual sensations, 138; *see also* basic awareness; direct awareness; introspective awareness

babies, 62, 74, 130
Baier, Kurt, 84–5, 85n1
barren sensations, 186, 187, 205–6
basic awareness, 117–18, 120, 131, 137
basic descriptions: semantic properties of, 175–8
behavior, 75–6; and ascribing sensations to other beings, 15; concepts standing for, 14; and distribution of sensations, 10; types of, 160
behaviorism, 12, 13, 44, 106
being a pain, 3, 65, 173–4, 183, 185, 215; errors of judgment about, 128–9; in functionalism, 81, 82, 235; identity with physical property, 99–100; infralinguistic concepts standing for, 163; in psychofunctionalism, 69; in type materialism, 97–8
being a sensation, 178–9, 181, 183, 185

being an itch, 3, 62–4; in functionalism, 235; infralinguistic concepts standing for, 163

belief(s), 85; awareness of sensation as, 119–20; cognitively spontaneous, 133–4; intentional content of, 144–7; *see also* introspective beliefs

belief-generating sensations, 186–7; awareness of, 187–206; and barren sensations, 205–6; diaphanous, 187; justification of beliefs about, 203–4

beliefs about sensations: concepts used in, 12–13; epistemological status of, 8, 108, 117–18, 126–30, 135; infallibility of, 12, 85, 107–8, 117, 127–9, 132; justification of, 131–7; of others, 9

Bentley, I.M., 123n6

best explanation principle, 41, 42; in ascription of sensations to others, 222, 225, 227; functionalism and, 48, 102; type materialism and, 22–6, 102

biological factors: in ascribing sensations to other beings, 15; in distribution of sensations, 10

biological function, 80

biological kind(s), 212, 214n4, 219

biological similarity, 106

biological species, 9, 209–17; ascription of psychological terms to, 54; ascription of sensations to, 77–80; distribution of mental states across, 45

biologically essential role(s): of conscious experience, 212, 219

Bisiach, E., 107n17

Black, Carolyn, 117n

Block, Ned, 44n, 47n3, 57–8, 57n10, 59, 59n11, 69n13, 101n14, 104, 104n15, 141n1

Blockean homunculi-heads, 57–8, 59, 68, 69n13, 70–3, 166; ascription of sensations to, 220, 221, 222; concept of pain and, 60–1

bodily sensations: awareness of, 193; concepts of, 159–85; concepts standing for, 160–1, 175; infralinguistic concepts of, 162–3; infratheoretical concepts of, 193–4; qualitative characteristics of, 210

BonJour, Laurence, 133–4, 133n12, 134n13

bounds of sense, 209, 224

Boyd, Richard N., 101n14

brain(s), 71, 166, 220, 222, 225; neurophysiological accounts of, 87

brain bisection, 230–1

brain-process theory, 26–7

brain processes: awareness of, 95–7; conscious experiences and, 24–5; interaction with sensations, 41–2; qualitative events and, 103–4

Broadbent, Donald E., 123n7

Brueckner, Anthony, 117n, 142n3, 143n5

Budd, Malcolm, 131, 131n11

C4PO, 71–3, 169

Carnap, Rudolf, 240–1, 240n6

Carpenter, Malcolm, 179n11

Cartesian argument, 6–7, 90–3, 94

Cartesian property, 48

Cartesianism, 12–13, 111, 204

causal roles, 14–15, 41–2, 159, 160, 162; of pain, 74, 79–80; state-types, 46; of tacit beliefs, 192–3

Causey, Robert L., 23n5, 25, 25n6

certainty, 85

Chisholm, Roderick M., 201, 201n6

Churchland, Paul, 53, 53n8, 88n3, 213, 213n3

closed-eye sensations, 186, 205–6

co-consciousness, 228, 229, 230, 231–2, 233, 234, 236, 237; direct awareness, 239–40

cognitive access: to visual sensations, 186

cognitive mechanism(s), 136; impaired, 150–1; relations between, 130

cognitive psychology, 55, 123n7

cognitively spontaneous beliefs, 133–4

Cohen, Stewart, 136n16, 143n4

color, 195–6

commonsense sensation terms: reference of, fixed by folk-psychological descriptions, 167–70; as synonymous with folk-psychological descriptions, 165–7, 181–2

compositional relations, 224, 228

conceivability, 60, 94–5, 180; as test for logical possibility, 90, 93–4

concept of pain, 8–9, 14, 61, 97–8, 137, 161; derivation of, 213, 214–15; generic, 217; intentional concept of, 144–7; skepticism and, 144–5

concept of sensation, 83–4, 137, 161, 178–83, 194

concepts: kinds of, 14; *see also* sensory concepts

concepts of bodily sensations: semantic properties of, 159–85

conceptual truths, 59–60, 67, 91, 92
Conee, Earl, 146n5, 167n5
conjunction law (probability calculus), 31–3, 36–7, 38
conscious experience: biologically essential role of, 212, 219; and brain process, 24–5; of other beings, 106
consciousness, 58, 117–18; whole states of, 240–3; *see also* unity of consciousness
conservatism, 102, 103, 104
contents, 159–61, 180–1; of belief-generating sensations, 199–204; of sensation concepts, 8–9, 159–60; theories of, 161, 164–78; of visual sensation concepts, 186–206
Copi, Irving M., 219, 219n12
core component, 79–80
correlation theses, 10, 12, 24, 25; functionalism, 48
correspondence relationship: between qualitative characteristics and physical characteristics, 405
co-spatial sensations, 237–8
counterpossibility principle, 143, 152–3; second, 149–50, 153

Dancy, Jonathan, 212–13, 213n2
Dark, Veronica J., 123n7
Davidson, Donald, 20n2
Davies, D.R., 123n7
Davis, Larry, 141n1
degree of internal articulation, 120, 121
demon hypothesis, 13, 141–2, 145, 146–8, 150–1, 153; rejection of, 147–8, 149
denial of sensations to other beings, 209–10, 224–5, 227
Dennett, D.C., 107n17, 108–14, 108n18, 109nn19, 20, 111n21, 112n22, 120n3
dependency relationship: between qualitative characteristics and physical characteristics, 4–5
Descartes, René, 84, 126, 136
description(s): fixing reference, 15, 167, 169, 170, 176, 181; and modal context(s), 177–8; names synonymous with folk-psychological, 164, 165–7, 169; normal form of, 171–2; *see also* folk-psychological descriptions
difference thresholds, 129n10
direct awareness, 188–9, 193, 194, 204; of belief-generating sensations, 187; as

co-conscious, 239; qualia accessible to, 210; of visual sensations, 198–9
direct awareness thesis, 130, 137–8, 140
direct realism, 188–9, 194, 195
discernibility condition, 149–50, 152, 155
double-aspect theory, 19–43, 44, 83; components of, 21; correlation thesis and, 25–6; and simplicity argument, 29–43
dreaming, 186, 194–5
Dretske, Fred, 143n4, 182n12
dual criterion theory, 176–8, 183
dualism, 44, 83, 169; arguments for, 84–95; content of, 20–1; correlation thesis and, 24–5; failings of, 19–43; epistemological arguments and, 84–7; functionalism and, 48; objections to type materialism and, 21–2; sensation terms and, 49; sensory events and, 6–7; and simplicity argument, 29–43

elementarerlebnisse, 240–1
eliminative materialism, 44, 106–14
empiricism, 204
entertaining appearances, 190–1, 192, 193, 200, 201, 203n10
epiphenomenalism, 26–7
epistemic safety, 36, 37
epistemological arguments, 65–7, 84–7; second, 80–2
epistemological questions, 7–8, 12–13; about other minds, 15–16
equipotentiality argument, 105, 106
errors, 128–30; of ignorance, 128–9; of judgment, 128–30
ersatz pain, 141–2, 144–5, 146, 149, 154–5
evidence, 112–13, 143, 149; for beliefs about sensations, 132; introspective, 147, 149, 152–3, 155; sensory, 118, 148, 149
exclusion principle: strong, 153–4; weak, 152–3, 155
experience: derivation of sensory concepts from, 212, 214–16; of pain, 147–8; qualitative aspects of, 87, 88–9; *see also* conscious experience
explanatory power, 42, 102; of hypotheses, 22; of materialism, 23n5, 27; of type materialism, 20, 25–6
extended synchronic p-spatial proximity, 238
externalist theories of meaning, 164–5

247

extramental entities, 127; attending to, 119, 123n7; awareness of, 194–7; concepts of, 195

extramental states of affairs: perception of, 188–9

Feigl, Herbert, 19n1
fetuses, 62, 74
Fetzer, James H., 27n8
first heterogeneity argument (psychofunctionalism), 73–6
first-person ascriptions, 135, 161, 182; justification of, 164–5, 166, 170; of pain, 81–2, 170
Fodor, Jerry, 39n15, 104, 104n15, 226n16
folk-psychological descriptions: commonsense sensation terms as synonymous with, 54–5, 165–7, 181–2; and nonimmediate sensations, 226–7; reference-fixing, 167, 169, 170, 181
folk psychology, 51n6, 53–5, 66, 106, 137, 162; axioms of, 182n12, 183; concepts of belief-generating sensations and, 200, 203; justification of beliefs in, 191, 193; laws of, 165, 226–7; vocabulary of, 72, 75, 221, 222
Forgus, Ronald H., 129n10
formal simplicity, 28, 29, 31–5, 41n16; value of, 33–4
foundationalism, 135n14, 202
Fox, Ivan, 83n, 117n, 121n4, 139n, 179n11, 228n, 240n6
Frege, Gottlob, 218, 218n11
functional organization, 59, 166, 231
functional properties, 47–8, 56, 80–1, 162; awareness of, 163; in Blockean androids, 70–1; correspondence with psychological theories, 50–6; distribution of sensations and, 10; functional role and, 167–9; identity of mental states with, 59–60; and internal states, 79–80; names referring to, 54–6, 69–70, 165; paradigmatic, 50; and qualitative characteristics, 61–7, 74–5; shared by sensations, 178–9, 181–2
functional relations, 239; in unity of consciousness, 234–5
functional role(s), 46–8, 56n9, 75–6, 170, 175, 182–3; contingency of, 177; functional properties and, 167–9; of mental states, 79–80; of neural state-types, 227; of pain, 146, 147, 154–5, 183

functionalism, 3n1, 7, 21, 105, 166; arguments for, 48–50; core doctrine of, 53, 55, 56; failings of, 19, 44–82, 83; forms of, 50, 53–6; and mental states, 45–50; multiple realization argument, 101–3; objections to, 56–82; skeptical argument in defense of, 154–5; theory of self in, 217n10; and theory of semantic properties of sensation concepts, 161; of qualitative states, 146–7; unity of consciousness in, 233–5

generalization from a single case, 213, 217–19
genericness: sensation concepts, 160–1, 175, 178, 181, 183
gestalten, 121
Goldman, Alvin I., 135–6, 135n15, 136n16
Goodman, Nelson, 33–4, 33n9, 34n10
Gosse, Philip, 26, 27
gustatory awareness, 189
gustatory sensations, 34; concepts standing for, 160–1, 175, 178; infralinguistic concepts of, 162–3; qualitative characteristics of, 210

Haldane, John, 131n11
hallucination, 186, 194–5, 201
Hardin, Clyde L., 39n15, 196n3
Harman, Gilbert, 22, 22n3, 188, 188n1
Hazen, Allan, 83n
heat, 161
Hellman, Geoffrey, 42–3, 42n17, 43n18
heterogeneity arguments: first, 73–6; second, 76–80
Hirsch, Eli, 242n7
human beings: similarity of sensations in, 209, 210, 212
Hume, David, 23n4, 214, 214n5, 217, 217n10
Hyslop, Alec, 214n4

identity propositions/statements, 92n5, 94, 95n9
immediate qualia (sensations), 209, 210, 219; ascription to remote species, 224; and neural state-types, 224–5
imperialism, 124–6
implicit definition theory, 14; alternatives to, 14–15
indexical beliefs, 146–7
indirect awareness, 188–9, 194
individuation, 241–3

inductive inference, 22–3, 28–40, 211–19
infallibility thesis, 127–9, 130
inferential awareness, 187, 193
information-processing mechanisms, 122, 123n7
infralinguistic (infratheoretical) sensation concepts, 161–3, 177, 180–1, 184n13, 185, 187, 194–5
inner eye hypothesis, 12, 119–20, 123–4, 125
inner vision, 118–20, 121, 123–6
intensity, 120–1
internal ostensive definitions, 8, 159, 180–1; sensory concepts get contents from, 14
internal scanning device, 7–8, 13, 119–20, 121, 125, 126
internal states, 61, 125, 160, 167–9; ascribing sensation terms to, 166; functional role of, 75–6, 78; in justification of first-person ascriptions, 170; misclassification of, 151; similarity among, in beings of same type, 219n14
intrinsic qualities, 3n1, 21, 80, 81, 210; and visual sensations, 197–8, 203–4, 205
introspectible changes, 125–6
introspection, 8, 12–13, 81, 107, 179, 180, 181, 184–5; and direct awareness, 204; in eliminative materialism, 109, 110, fallibility of, 107, 108, 117; and the skeptic, 139–55; theory of, 82, 117, 127; two-factor theory of, 13; in understanding of p-spatial relations, 237; views of, 131–7
introspectionist tradition, 122n6, 161
introspective awareness, 50, 117–38, 147; nature of, 7–0; of self, 214; sensory concepts derived from, 214–15; theory of, 108; and unity of consciousness, 231–3
introspective beliefs, 126–30; certainty of, 8; differ from perceptual beliefs, 127; epistemological status of, 160; justification of, 117, 131–7, 204; justification of skepticism about, 139–42, 143–4, 147–55
irreducibly mental properties, 98
irreducibility, 38, 39n15
itching, 62, 64, 65, 75, 161, 173n10; linguistic concept of, 164; see also *being an itch*

Jackson, Frank, 201n6, 214n4
Jacoby, Henry, 83n, 167n5, 173n10

James, William, 8, 122n6
Johnston, William A., 123n7
judgment: errors of, 127, 128–30; about qualitative states, 111, 112, 113–14
justification(s), 65, 66–7, 153–4, 193; of ascription of pain, 81–2; of ascription of sensations to others, 209–11, 214–28; of ascription of sensations to remote species, 209, 222–4; for belief in folk psychology, 191; of beliefs about belief-generating sensations, 203–4; of first-person ascriptions, 164–5, 166, 170; of visual beliefs, 200–2

Kahneman, Daniel, 123n7
Kim, Jaegwon, 106, 106n16
kind-term/concept, 145
Kirk, Robert, 83n
Kitcher, Philip, 23n4
knowledge, 85; of other minds, 207–27
Kripke, Saul A., 15, 15n3, 91, 91n4, 93n6, 94n8, 215–17, 215n8, 217n10

Lee, Richard, 44n
Leibniz, Gottfried von, 24
Leibniz's law, 85, 86, 88
Levin, Michael, 164, 164n1, 167n5
Levine, Joseph, 139n, 228n
Lewis, David, 11n2, 47n3
Loar, Brian, 47n2, 51n7, 56n9
logical necessity (criterion of), 91–3
logical possibility, 67, 68, 229; conceivability as test for, 90, 93–4; and ersatz pain, 141
look-sustaining states, 201–4
lower organisms: sensations in, 167, 179–80; *see also* remote species
Lycan, William G., 22, 22n3, 23n5, 69n13, 83n, 98n12, 117n, 124n8, 167n5

McDowell, John, 142n3
Malcolm, Norman, 214–15, 214n6, 216, 217n10
manifest nature thesis, 130, 137–8
Marcel, A.J., 107n17
Marsh, R.C., 36n13
material objects, 36–7
materialism, 19–20; explanatory power of, 23n5, 27; forms of, 11–12; sensory events in, 6–7
mathematical simplicity, 28–9, 41n16
Melamed, Lawrence E., 129n10

memory: in eliminative materialism, 109,
110, 113–14; fallibility of, 108
mental states, 20, 75–6; awareness of, 95–
7; functional role of, 79–80;
functionalism and, 45–50; identity with
functional properties, 59–60
Mill, John Stuart, 211, 211n1
Miller, Richard W., 41n16
mind–body problem, 7, 12, 98, 140–1;
type materialism as answer to, 24
minimal interpretation, 68–9
modes of presentation, 98–101
multiple realization argument, 101–3,
104
Munitz, Milton K., 91n4

Nagel, Thomas, 87–8, 87n2, 89–90
names: sensation terms, 164–5, 168, 169,
174, 175; strictly rigid, 178, 181;
synonymous with folk-psychological
descriptions, 165–7
natural kind words, 170–5
natural kinds, 105, 106, 219
neighboring species: nonimmediate
sensations in, 226–7; *see also* biological
species; other beings
Nelson, R.J., 83n
neural relations: between sensations, 238–
40
neurological characteristics: qualitative
characteristics and, 11–12, 96–8, 101–3
neurological equipotentiality (Lashleyan
doctrine of), 104
Nisbett, R.E., 219n13
Nissen, Lowell, 44n
nomological (physical) possibility, 67, 68,
69; of locationless sensations, 180;
unity relations, 235
nomological danglers, 19n1
nonbiological beings: ascription of
mental states to, 45; *see also* androids;
remote species
nondoxastic foundationalism, 202
nondoxastic internalism, 134n14
nonimmediate qualia/sensations, 210,
225–7
nonrigid designator(s), 178
numbers, 36, 37–8

Ockham's Razor, 35–6, 38, 39–40
olfactory sensations, 3; concepts standing
for, 160–1, 175, 178; infralinguistic
concepts of, 162–3; qualitative

characteristics of, 210; semantic
properties of, 183–5
ontological simplicity, 28, 29, 35–40, 41n6
other beings: ascription of sensations to,
54, 57–9, 60–1, 68, 69–73, 77–80;
conscious experience of, 106; denial of
sensations to, 209–10, 224–5, 227;
internal states, 169; intuitions about
sensations in, 166, 167, 210; *see also*
androids; Blockean homunculi-heads;
remote species
other minds: knowledge of, 207–27;
otherness of, 16; questions about, 9, 15–
16; unity of consciousness and, 228–9
other minds problem, 209–11; argument
from analogy (AA), 211–19; in
synthetic folk psychologism, 167
otherness, 9, 16

p-spatial relations, 236–8, 239
pain: in animal species, 77, 78, 79–80;
ascription to other beings, 72–3;
awareness of, 147, 191, 231–2;
biological function of, 80; capacity to
experience, 146–7, 151, 235;
conceivability of, 90; distribution of, 5;
functional role of, 154–5; in
functionalism, 45, 46, 48, 58–9, 60–1,
65–6, 69, 78–80; infralinguistic concept
of, 161–2; introspective beliefs about,
204; justification of beliefs about, 131–
2, 141–8, 149–51, 152–5; linguistic
concepts of, 161, 164; natural kind
words for, 170; in psychofunctionalism,
72, 73, 75, 76; role played by, in
human beings, 77; in synthetic folk-
psychologism, 167, 168–9; vector for,
173–5, 183; *see also being a pain*; concept
of pain; ersatz pain
Pappas, G.S., 135n15
paralysis victims, 62, 74
Parasuraman, Raja, 123n7
Parfit, Derek, 230–1, 230n1, 240
parsimony (principle), 26, 27
part–whole relations, 235–6
Peacocke, Christopher, 197–9, 197n4,
198n5
Peano postulates, 33, 34
perception, 118, 189; sense, 139–42, 144;
see also representational theory of
perception; visual perception
perceptual awareness: different from
introspective awareness, 118

perceptual beliefs, 136, 186–7; different
from introspective beliefs, 127;
propositions representing, 139–40, 148
perceptual model(s), 124
Perkins, Moreland, 196n2
Pettit, Philip, 142n3
phenomenal similarity relation, 185, 195–
6, 237
phenomenal space, 228–43; auditory
sensations in, 236; location of
sensations in, 179–80
phenomenalism, 204
physical characteristics: relationship with
qualitative characteristics, 4–5, 11–12,
21
physical events: relationship with sensory
events, 6–7, 11–12, 20–1
physical state-types, 45–6, 169
physical states: sensory states and, 84–90,
97–8
pictorial depth cues, 206
Pillsbury, W.B., 122nn5, 6
Pollock, John L., 135n14, 202n7
Popper, Sir Karl, 41n16
possible worlds, 67, 92n5, 169, 178
principle of physical exhaustion, 42–3
principles of entification, 241–2, 243
probability calculus: conjunction law of,
31–3, 36–7, 38
probability of truth, 36–7, 136
prominence, 120, 122n5, 123n6
proper individual(s), 241–3
property dualism argument, 98–9, 100, 101
propositional attitudes, 44, 52n7, 88, 162;
verbs of, 85–6
psychofunctionalism, 55–6, 166;
objections to, 57, 67–82
psychological properties, 55, 56, 69; first/
second order, 47, 48; and functional
roles, 46–7; identical with functional
properties, 47–8, 60
psychological states: of Blockean
homunculi, 58; relation to other
psychological states, 76–7, 78–9; in
visual perception, 190–1
psychological terms, 69–70, 164–85; in
folk psychology, 53–4; semantic
properties of, 53; and truth of
functionalism, 49–50, 55–6
psychological theories: functional
properties' correspondence with, 50–6
psychophysical correlation thesis, 10, 11–
12, 21, 23–4

psychophysical correlations, 104
psychophysical laws: in dualism, 27;
explanations of, 25; synchronic/
diachronic, 30, 32
psychophysics, 224
purely sensory relations, 228
Putnam, Hilary, 45n1, 142n3, 170–5,
171n8, 172n9, 183

qualia, 3, 4, 52n7, 111, 113; identity with
physical characteristics, 7; kinds of,
210; *see also* immediate qualia
(sensations)
qualitative awareness, 137–8
qualitative characteristics, 3–4, 8, 11, 162,
165, 178–9, 182, 185, 210; correlation
theses, 10, 12; and functional
properties, 61–7, 74–5; in
functionalism, 50; immediate quale,
209; as intrinsic characteristics, 21;
metaphysical nature of, 44; and
neurological characteristics, 96–8, 101–
3; of pain, 147, 154–5; recognition of,
163; relationship with physical
characteristics, 4–5, 11–12, 21; ultimate
nature of, 7; *see also* qualia
qualitative concepts, 137
quasi-empirical questions, 4–5, 9–11, 13
quasifunctional properties, 49–50

Railton, Peter, 22n4
Ramsey, F.P., 52
Ramsey functional correlates, 52, 53, 55
Ramsey functional descriptions, 52–3, 54–
5, 56n9, 66, 165
Ramsey sentence, 182n12, 183
reactive dispositions, 112, 113–14
reduction(s), 24n5, 42, 46
reference-fixing, 15; by folk-
psychological descriptions, 167, 169,
170, 176, 181; indeterminacy of, 168; of
term "sensation," 182–3
relations: causal, 235; concepts of, 214; *p*-
spatial, 236–8; part–whole, 235–6;
sources/forms of unity of
consciousness, 228, 229, 233, 234, 238–
43
relevant alternatives, 143–4
reliabilism, 136
reliability condition, 218, 219
remote species: ascription of sensations
to, 209–11, 220–4; denial of sensations
in, 209–10, 224–5

representational theory of perception, 188–9, 194, 196
Resnik, Michael, 19n
rigid designator(s), 94n8, 178
Roach, David, 117n
Rosenthal, David, 27n7, 49n4
Russell, Bertrand, 35–6, 35n11, 36nn12, 13, 38, 39, 39n14

Salmon, Wesley C., 23n4
sample size: and argument from analogy, 213, 217–19
Schiffer, Stephen, 51n7
Schroeder, David A., 117n
second absent qualia argument, 70–3, 77–8
second counterpossibility principle, 149–50
second epistemological argument, 80–2
second heterogeneity argument, 76–80
Selby-Bigge, L.A., 214n5
selective confirmation, 143, 149, 152–3, 155
self, 44; concept of, 216, 217; introspective awareness of, 214, 217
self-intimation thesis, 127–8, 129–30
Sellars, Wilfrid, 22, 22n3
semantic complaint (psychofunctionalism), 69–70
semantic marker(s), 170–5
semantic properties: of concepts of bodily sensations, 159–85; of visual sensation concepts, 186, 187
semantic questions, 8–9, 13–15
Senor, Thomas, 117n, 136n16
sensation: concept of, 83–4, 137, 161, 178–83, 194
sensation concepts; see concepts of bodily sensations; sensory concepts
sensation of heat, 175–8, 185
sensation terms, 49; and ascription of sensations to others, 221–2; as descriptions/as names, 167–70; theories of meaning for, 164–78; vectors for, 174–5, 183
sensations, 3, 13, 106; activation of, 121–2; ascription to animal species, 77–80; distribution of, 5, 10, 74–5, 76, 166; epistemic access to, 12–13; experience of, 87–9 (see also sense experience); extension of notion of, to others, 216; individual, 240–1; infallibility/omniscience regarding, 8, 12, 13;

introspective awareness of, 117–38; in justification of beliefs about sensations, 131–7; metaphysical nature of, 6–7, 11–12, 44; neural relations between, 238–40; phenomenological nature of, 159; as proper individuals, 241–3; realist attitude toward, 83–4, 106–7; simultaneous, 240; unextended, 242–3; unity of, 231–3
sensory beliefs; see beliefs about sensations
sensory concepts: and concepts of causal roles, 14–15; contents of, 8–9, 14; derived from introspective awareness, 214–15; in eliminative materialism, 106–14; ostensive, 14, 15
sensory events, 6–7, 38; relationship with physical events, 6–7, 11–12, 20–1
sensory field, 16, 232–3
sensory relations: and relations of physical objects in physical space, 236–8
set theory, 36, 37, 39n14
Sextus Empiricus, 136
Shaffer, Jerome, 95n10, 98n12
Shoemaker, Sydney, 44n, 83n, 117n, 139n, 141n2, 154n6, 159n, 167n5, 186n, 233–4, 233n4
similarity(ies): and ascription of sensations to others, 218, 219, 220–1, 222, 223, 224, 226–7; between other beings and ourselves, 166; of sensations in human beings, 209, 210, 212, 219n14; structural, 224
similarity relations, 185, 195–6, 237; qualitative, 180–1
simplicity, 26, 27, 42, 102, 103, 104, 113, 126; forms of, 28–9; mathematical, 28–9, 41n16; of type materialism, 20; see also formal simplicity; ontological simplicity
simplicity argument: justifying materialism, 26–9; justifying type materialism, 29–43
skepticism, 13, 23n4, 136–7, 191; introspection and, 139–55; justification of, 139–42, 143–4, 147–55
Smart, J.J.C., 19, 20 23n5, 26–7, 27nn7,8, 49, 49nn4, 5, 164n1
Sober, Elliott, 40n16
spatial part–whole relations, 235
spectrum inversion, 69n13, 197
Squires, Roger, 131n11

state-tokens, 105, 165; ascription of
   sensation to internal, 181, 184–5; in
   functionalism, 64, 65, 66, 67–8; neural/
   sensory, 30, 32
state-type(s), 32, 43, 165, 174–5, 182;
   functional role of, 168–9; in
   functionalism, 45, 46, 47, 48, 51–2,
   56n7, 64, 65, 67; immediate qualia and,
   225; infralinguistic concepts for, 185;
   in lower organisms, 167; internal, 167–
   9; neural, 30, 45, 224–5, 227
states of awareness, 118, 137–8, 151
Stephens, Lynn, 83n, 186n
stereoscopic fallacy, 98n12
stereotype(s), 170–5, 183
Stevenson, Leslie, 131n11
strong exclusion principle, 153–4
strong equivalence, 91–2
Swinburne, Richard, 233n4
synchronic unity, 233–4
syntactic marker(s), 170–5
synthetic folk psychologism, 167–70
systematization, 33–4

Thagaard, P., 219n13
Thompson, Frank W., 42–3, 42n17, 43n18
Titchener, Edward B., 122n6
token materialism, 11, 20, 84, 87–8
transtemporal similarity judgments, 108
Triesman, Anne, 123n7
Truex, Raymond, 179n11
type materialism, 11–12, 44, 159–60; as
   answer to mind–body problem, 24;
   defense of, 19, 57, 83–114; explanatory
   power of, 20, 25–6; implicit definition
   theory incompatible with, 14; objections
   to, 83–114; and other minds, 211;
   semantic issues in, 13–14, 15; simplicity
   argument justifying, 29–43; superiority
   of, to dualism and double-aspect theory,
   20–6, 27–9; truth of, 23, 95–8

unconscious sensation(s), 118
unity of consciousness, 9, 16, 228–43;
   analysis of, in terms of ownership,
   229–31; functionalist theory of, 233–5;
   introspective awareness in, 231–3;
   relations as source of, 240–3; sources/
   forms of, 228, 229, 233, 234, 238–40
unity relations, 228, 229, 233, 234–5, 237,
   239; extended synchronic p-spatial
   proximity as, 238; "ghostly," 239–40
universal correlation, 5, 11
universals, 11n2, 163, 169; natural kind
   words standing for, 170
unlocated sensations, 179–80

van Fraassen, Bas C., 23n4
vector(s) (Putnamian), 171–5, 183
verb(s), 170; of propositional attitudes,
   85–6
veridical visual perception, 186, 194
visual appearance(s): entertaining, 190–1,
   192, 193
visual awareness: forms of, 194
visual belief(s), 200–2
visual perception, 187–94, 204;
   psychological states in, 190–1
visual sensations, 231–2; awareness of,
   138, 193–4; concepts of, 186–206;
   existence of, 191–4; qualitative
   characteristics of, 210; types of, 186
volume adjustment, 13, 118, 120–1, 123,
   126
Vries, Willem de, 83n, 117n

weak exclusion principle, 152–3, 155
Westendorf, David, 117n, 228n
White, Stephen, 83n, 98–9, 99n13, 100
William of Ockham, 35
Wilson, Mark, 39n15
Wittgenstein, Ludwig, 131–2, 161
Wundt, Wilhelm, 122n6